SECRET SUFFERING

How Women's Sexual and Pelvic Pain Affects Their Relationships

Susan Bilheimer and Robert J. Echenberg, MD

Foreword by Daniel Brookoff, MD, PhD

Sex, Love, and Psychology
Judy Kuriansky, Series Editor

PRAEGER
An Imprint of ABC-CLIO, LLC

A B C CLIO

Santa Barbara, California • Denver, Colorado • Oxford, England

Library of Congress Cataloging-in-Publication Data

Bilheimer, Susan.
Secret suffering : how women's sexual and pelvic pain affects their relationships / Susan Bilheimer and Robert J. Echenberg ; foreword by Daniel Brookoff.
    p. cm. — (Sex, love, and psychology)
   Includes bibliographical references and index.
    ISBN 978-0-313-35921-7 (alk. paper) — ISBN 978-0-313-35922-4 (ebook : alk. paper) 1. Dyspareunia—Pathophysiology. 2. Pelvic pain—Pathophysiology.
3. Dyspareunia—Psychological aspects. 4. Pelvic pain—Psychological aspects. 5. Women—Diseases. 6. Intimacy (Psychology) I. Echenberg, Robert J. II. Title.
RC560.D97B55 2009
616.7'1—dc22   2009009845

13   12   11   10   9   1   2   3   4   5

This book is also available on the World Wide Web as an eBook.
Visit www.abc-clio.com for details.

ABC-CLIO, LLC
130 Cremona Drive, P.O. Box 1911
Santa Barbara, California 93116-1911

This book is printed on acid-free paper ∞
Manufactured in the United States of America

This book is for general information only. No book can ever substitute for the judgment of a medical professional. If you have worries or concerns, contact your doctor. The names and many details of individuals discussed in this book have been changed to protect the patients' identities.

Some of the stories are composites of patient interactions created for illustrative purposes.

CONTENTS

FOREWORD: WHAT DO *I* KNOW?

I have been providing medical care for people with chronic pelvic and sexual pain for nearly 30 years. One thing I know is that people with chronic pelvic pain are some of the strongest, most courageous, and kindest people that I have ever met. Though they often don't feel heroic, they truly are my heroes. In this book, Susan Bilheimer and Dr. Robert J. Echenberg share stories of heroic people who have kept on going despite a level of pain and suffering that has sometimes approached the unbelievable, but always true.

It is interesting to note that the title of this book about people with sexual and pelvic pain actually addresses the suffering before pain. That is because pain is something that happens to a body, while suffering is something that happens to a person. As Hippocrates himself taught us, it is the suffering person that physicians must face, not just the pain.

So what do *I* know? I used to think I knew a whole lot. I would spend a great deal of time explaining things to people whose suffering I faced. But as I grew older, I realized that I really knew less and less. I started spending less time talking and more time listening. I started to understand what Hippocrates taught when he said "a patient has an obligation to disclose and describe his pain. It is the patient's duty to relate accurately what he has experienced and the physician's duty to listen."

One of the most important things that a person who is living in turmoil can do is to seek and find peace. Find and embrace the people who comfort you and bring you closer to peace, and let go of those who take you in the other direction.

It is our job as physicians to help pelvic and sexual pain patients recover physically. But it is also our duty to listen, treat them with respect and dignity, and do all we can to make it easier for them to find that peace.

For thousands of years, one way we have taken care of each other and shown each other that we are not alone in times of crisis has been to tell each other stories about heroes. Though these stories may not relieve physical pain, they join our hopes and our strengths together and help us alleviate suffering. And they almost always help us find solutions for the worst pain of all, the pain of hopelessness and abandonment.

Secret Suffering is a clarion call to the medical community to take heed of this message and, through the stories of the heroes in this book, also provides a source of solace and support for both those who suffer and their partners.

Daniel Brookoff, MD, PhD

PREFACE

Women suffering from chronic pelvic pain (CPP) face two obstacles: dealing with their pain, whether emotional, physical, or spiritual; and understanding their pain medically and physiologically, its sources, causes, and manifestations. This important volume seeks to unite these approaches to CPP by offering insight on both medical and personal experiences to women suffering from this painful and life-disrupting affliction, their families, and their physicians.

Together, with my background as a physician and Susan's experience as a sexual pain sufferer, we hope to raise the consciousness of CPP sufferers, the general public, and the many health care providers who haven't been listening closely enough. Women, their loved ones, and physicians need to know how prevalent these disorders are; how they decimate relationships; and what physicians can do to recognize, address, and effectively treat these conditions.

Susan approaches this work from an experiential perspective. She has endured years of pain, humiliation, and guilt as a wife who felt she was not able to fulfill the loving and tender sexual needs of her husband. She quickly grew disillusioned with the medical profession as doctor after doctor misdiagnosed her and failed to find causes, let alone solutions, for her pain.

Susan and her husband, Jay, determined that their experiences with CPP needed to be shared with other sufferers and their loved ones in an attempt to help other misunderstood and misdiagnosed women. Susan boldly stepped up to the plate; she has undergone quite a journey in preparation for this volume, interviewing and collecting the stories of women (and men) who suffer from CPP and their partners with the purpose of helping CPP sufferers understand they are not alone and should not stay silent any longer. Susan's other purpose in writing *Secret Suffering* is to provide public exposure of this devastating issue so that the medical community will finally validate and legitimize CPP and physicians will take appropriate measures to avoid misdiagnosis and appropriately treat patients so they can successfully manage their condition.

I was delighted to help Susan achieve this aim and also to contribute to this volume the medical perspective necessary to help women and their physicians begin to understand the physicality of CPP and to improve patient quality of life, which is of paramount importance. When my patients are able to lead lives that are more normal and have improved relationships at home, in the bedroom, at work, and at school, they are among the most grateful patients I have ever treated in decades as a gynecologist and obstetrician.

My OB/GYN career began in 1970. By the new millennium, I was no longer practicing obstetrics. I worked in a hospital setting, and in 2001, the chief of our department asked me to establish a CPP program that would focus on a *nonsurgical* approach to assessment and management. We based this new modality on findings that a significant percentage of diagnostic laparoscopies and other invasive and costly diagnostic studies traditionally yielded either negative or minimally positive findings. These findings did not explain the pathophysiology of noncyclic, chronic female pelvic pain.

Having spent over 30 years as a gynecologist, I believed that at least 70 to 80 percent of CPP was due to pelvic endometriosis and that ovarian cysts, pelvic adhesions, and pelvic inflammatory disease rounded out the remaining 20 to 30 percent. However, I became increasingly frustrated as I performed surgeries and did exhaustive testing on so many healthy-appearing young women and was still coming away unable to adequately diagnose and treat the origins of their pain. Thus began my journey toward specializing in CPP.

I saw my first severe CPP patients in a small examining room in the hospital's general pain management center. Working closely with a pain specialist/anesthesiologist was especially helpful in those early months. He gave me pointers on the medical management of chronic pain in general and was pleased to see my intense interest in treating pelvic pain. He reminded me that his training and specialization did not include CPP. I have since discovered that's true for most pain management specialists.

It became apparent that I knew almost nothing about the difference between acute and chronic pain. In medical school, we were taught the acute pain model, which all too often is our only tool in dealing with chronic pain in women.

If evidence of acute tissue damage was not visually documented through either surgical or radiological means, and the patient's subjective account of pain far exceeded the findings, then her symptoms were either disregarded, discounted, or minimized. Worse, she might have been looked upon as hysterical or as psychologically or emotionally unbalanced. The sad fact is that this view persists today. As evidence of this misguided thinking, I recently spoke to a group of physicians, and before beginning my talk, I was asked how I could tolerate caring for so many women who must be "hysterical drug seekers."

How wrong we have all been. Through my study and experience, I learned that, in fact, multiple diagnoses are common within CPP.[1]

In 2006, I opened my own practice, specializing in CPP. In some cases, I saw young women under 25 who had been through 7 or 8 laparoscopies and even hysterectomies. Even more tragic was knowing that, by the time I saw them, their pain was worse than ever.

My patients' relationships suffered tremendously. Depression, anxiety, frustration, and anger commonly appeared. Their distrust of the medical system was already significant, which meant I needed to show a great deal of concern to begin the healing process.

Working with CPP patients, I realized that I was not curing, but caring, and significantly improving the quality of life of most of these women. Many patients asserted that simply being heard, believed, and validated in their pain contributed to feeling better for the first time in months, years, and even decades.

The sexual health and quality of life for so many women and their partners depend on educating the medical community and changing their attitude toward CPP patients. The secret suffering must end, and Susan and I hope that this volume will contribute to increased and productive understanding of CPP, from both emotional and medical standpoints, among women and the physicians who treat them.

Robert J. Echenberg, MD, FACOG
December 2008

ACKNOWLEDGMENTS

From Susan Bilheimer

This book is a fulfillment of a dream for me. I need to thank the three women who made publication of *Secret Suffering* possible. Marjorie Veiga, who was the marketing director of the National Vulvodynia Association, pushed me to contact Dr. Judy Kuriansky because she thought she might be interested in participating in this project as a subject expert. Dr. Kuriansky, who is also a series editor for Praeger Publishers, was not only interested in being interviewed, but passed on our proposal for consideration to the publisher. Debbie Carvalko, the Senior Acquisitions Editor, psychology, health, and social work for Praeger, facilitated our book's acceptance and has patiently answered my many, many questions over the past year.

Thanks to Janet T. Przybylowicz for her incredibly nimble fingers (which transcribed hours and hours of taped interviews) and for her ability to keep me from being a complete administrative disaster. My appreciation goes out, as well, to Dr. Echenberg's wife, Nancy, for her detailed editing and continued support. In addition, thanks to Holly Monteith, technical editor, and Sara Kraus, illustrator, who came in at the last minute and pulled rabbits out of hats.

Finally, I am eternally grateful to the three most important people in my life because they made this project a reality for me. My husband, Jay, encouraged me to write this book for a year before I found the courage to do so. He loved me enough to allow me to lay bare the most intimate details of our life without complaint and has been my editorial sounding board throughout the process. Laura Paliganoff, my best friend, had the unsavory job of continually whipping me into shape each time I experienced a meltdown and thought this book would never come together. And my 18-year-old son, Sam, who finally stopped running out of the room at the mere mention of the subject matter of *Secret Suffering*, helped me organize the material, gave me pep talks on a regular basis, and simply said, "Go write your book," whenever I nagged him to clean his room, which turned out to be sage advice.

From Dr. Echenberg

Janet T. Przybylowicz and Sandy DiDona have been invaluable in helping me establish a private practice approach to chronic pelvic pain. As office and clinical managers, they have tirelessly worked to invent the wheel in today's harsh health care environment and allowed us all to develop a successful, profitable, and unique program when, I believe, many others thought it to be impossible.

I would like to acknowledge Kristin Fenstermaker and Melissa Sule, the rest of my staff, for the dedication, compassion, and professionalism that they have shared with our patients. The entire staff has made our office a safe haven for those who have otherwise lost trust in the system and even in themselves.

Also my thanks goes out to Dr. Alan Brau, Barbara and Keith DelPrete, and Lisa Cohan for giving me so much help and encouragement to overcome my reluctance and fears and move forward to develop my own program for pelvic pain. And finally, gratitude to the many nonphysician professionals and growing number of referring practitioners, all of whom have worked in conjunction with our program and have been such an integral part of improving the quality of life for so many of our patients.

And without a doubt, I truly cannot say enough about our patients themselves, many of whom have suffered so greatly and for so long but who have, indeed, inspired and taught us all, and for whom I will be eternally grateful. As for my loving wife, Nancy, I dedicate my portion of this work to her and can only express my devotion and everlasting love for her sacrifices and patience throughout our professional transitions and challenges over these past few years.

Finally, from both of us

We thank all the experts who spoke with us and gave us the words to guide our readers. And thank you to all the men and women who entrusted their very personal stories to us.

Chapter One

WHY THIS BOOK HAD TO BE WRITTEN

There is a tremendous stigma about the subject of sexual pain. It's so personal that you just don't talk about it. Nobody is out there talking about it like you would if you had, you know, other problems . . . like a bad hair day.

—Marcie (interviewee)

I wasn't prepared for the woman who told me that her pain had peaked so badly that as she watched that famous clip on TV of Saddam Hussein about to be executed, she actually envied him at that moment "because he was about to die."

—Robert J. Echenberg, MD

I became hysterical and when my husband got home I fell down on the floor and just begged him to kill me because I couldn't do my job, I couldn't be a wife, I couldn't take care of my child, and there was no reason for me to go on.

—Jane (interviewee)

Chronic sexual and pelvic pain is destroying the lives of millions of women and their families. The medical community is not doing enough to help them. Dr. Echenberg and I felt compelled to bring this staggering epidemic to light for all those who won't speak up for themselves and to give voice to women and men who don't want to stay silent any longer. Throughout this book, you'll read the stories of patients and their partners. You'll learn what it's like to live in their skin. You'll hear from top experts who are forging a new path to recovery.

Dr. Echenberg and I come to *Secret Suffering* from different perspectives. He has focused on treating women with sexual (and pelvic) pain for over eight years. I am a woman who has suffered with sexual pain for most of my adult life. Both of us believe with all our hearts that this destructive syndrome and its effects on relationships cannot stay hidden anymore, shrouded in shame and secrecy.

SUSAN'S STORY

My husband, Jay, and I were married in 2003. After a year, I began having consistent and increasing vaginal pain during intercourse. I'd had vaginal infections, or what I thought were infections, for decades. I'd been on one antibiotic after another for various "bugs" in my vagina: one week strep, the next e-coli, then bacterial vaginosis, and on and on.

My vagina never totally healed. And then, sex became torturous. Jay's penis felt like a hot poker scorching the skin of my vagina, a poker with sharp needles stabbing its sensitive walls. I loved him, and he loved me, but in some ways, making love felt like a self-inflicted rape. He wanted to have intercourse, but he didn't want to hurt me. I'd feel guilty and tell him to go ahead. Afterward, my insides felt as if they'd been torched. Sometimes, I could barely walk to the bathroom after sex. The burning ignited what seemed like my entire nervous system, sending out flames like hot tentacles, coursing through my body. I felt physically violated. Even a touch on my clitoris sometimes felt like pins sticking into me.

Too many times, I shoved my husband off me, pushing him out of me, imploring him between sobs to find someone else—a woman who could have "real" sex, who could *enjoy* sex.

Over the next few years, I saw doctor after doctor, with no help, no accurate diagnosis, and no helpful ideas. Oh, yes, I did uncover one invaluable piece of information. In 2005, an immunologist got me off the hamster wheel of antibiotics. The bottom line was that she said my overgrowths weren't true infections, and taking course after course of antibiotics only worsened my problem.

Once I stopped taking antibiotics, I watched my pain and burning ebb and flow. When I insisted doctors do cultures instead of pumping me full of antibiotics first, I found time after time that there was, indeed, no infection. Since seeing that immunologist nearly four years ago, I've only had two true vaginal infections. (However, I must note that while this is true for me, you must always see your health care practitioner to be examined and have a culture if you have symptoms leading you to believe you have an infection.)

I was angry and enraged at all the doctors I'd seen who dismissed my concerns when they saw nothing organically wrong, implied I was crazy, misdiagnosed me, or gave me a remedy that didn't help at all. Because of my experiences with the medical community and the harrowing journey we'd taken as a couple, winding our way through this mess, Jay encouraged me to write a book about the toll this horrifying problem takes on women and their partners. Write their stories for them, he urged, because this condition is as humiliating as it is painful and destructive. He said, "There must be other women who are like you, but keep the pain to themselves. Chances are they don't even tell their doctors. Be their voice. Say what they can't say. Give them hope."

"Not only the sufferers," continued Jay, "but the *partners* of these women might learn something from couples willing to speak out and share their stories." No way, I thought. Who on earth would want to read about my painful vagina, much less anyone else's?

But he continued prodding me, and a year after that conversation, I decided I had to write this book despite my trepidation because my own search for information about sexual pain conditions such as vulvodynia and interstitial cystitis lead me to other women's stories, women so frustrated they developed the courage to finally speak out. After reading each story, I found I could breathe better just thinking, "I'm not the only one. Other suffering women feel the same way." I knew then that there was healing in just knowing that I wasn't alone or crazy, and I felt certain that would be true for others as well.

MEETING DR. ECHENBERG

I approached Dr. Helene Leonetti, a gynecologist, who had contributed the foreword to a meditation book I wrote for midlife women. She put me in touch with Dr. Echenberg, the man who changed my life, a confidant, and the medical expert collaborator of this book.

I live in Florida, but there was no question we had to meet. So I went to Pennsylvania, watched how he and his staff worked, spoke with some of his patients, and had my own examination.

He spent the same amount of time with me as with any other new patient: two hours. I finally had a diagnosis, or rather, a crate full of them. All the confusion began to peel away like layers of an onion. My diagnoses are chronic pelvic pain (CPP), with the following specific conditions: pelvic floor dysfunction, pudendal neuralgia, vulvar vestibulitis, vulvodynia, and interstitial cystitis. I had no clue what half of these meant at the time. I already knew I had migraines and fibromyalgia, but now I learned that even these seemingly unrelated illnesses were also connected to my problems.

Most surprisingly, I realized that these symptoms are not just a middle-aged lady problem. They often start early in life, triggered by trauma or other negative events. They simmer in a memory bank within the central nervous system until they finally break through the surface of consciousness for some of us, often resulting in the collapse of relationships, divorce, job loss, depression, hopelessness, loss of dignity, and even thoughts of suicide.

Dr. Echenberg opened this Pandora's Box of issues for me, the same issues that are brewing in stories I've read on the Internet and interviews I conducted. Women with sexual pain want their quality of life back. They want their bodies healed and their sexuality brought back to life. They want their self-esteem renewed and their broken relationships restored.

Dr. Echenberg understood that, and I was thrilled and relieved. Despite the obstacles I faced, I could see light emerging. I wanted to share my experiences with other suffering women so that they, too, might see the light of hope by understanding their own pain through mine. To this end, you'll find my personal stories and reflections throughout the book in sections called "Living with CPP: Susan's Journal."

DEVELOPING THE PROJECT AND WRITING THE BOOK

I was overwhelmed with the number of women willing to come forward to speak about their rage, sadness, and frustration, to tell me their stories and share their pain. Well over 100 women and at least 20 partners contacted me. I gathered these potential interviewees from different sources, including an Internet survey I conducted (more details about the survey are contained in Appendix C).[1]

I believe that those who suffer from this condition merit the respect and common decency from the medical community that is provided to any patient. We deserve the validation that we have legitimate health issues and our pain is real. If doctors don't know how to properly diagnose and treat us, they should admit it and be willing to learn or know the appropriate specialist for referral.

The good news is that the secret of chronic sexual and pelvic pain suffered by millions of women is going public because patients and an increasing number of exceptional doctors and researchers will no longer stand for keeping our agony cloaked in silence and having the medical community ignore our pleas for help. Dr. Echenberg, my husband, and I fervently hope *Secret Suffering* contributes to this groundswell of support and healing.

Chapter Two

THE MANY FACES OF SEXUAL PAIN

I wake up pain-free every day, but it gradually builds throughout the day. The area where I burn is all external. Usually it feels like it's on fire, yet dry, like the gauze the dentist puts in my mouth. I found that ice packs can be my best friend. I put them right over my vagina.

—Lauren (interviewee)

It hurts upon penetration, and hurts increasingly more with thrusting, like my skin is wearing off.

—Survey respondent

This pain is unbearable and I only hope that we find a cure someday. It's depressing. Please help us. I'm only 25 and I've never had sex without pain. This is a sad reality.

—Survey respondent

What exactly is sexual pain? There are as many variations as there are those who suffer from this debilitating affliction. Some women describe it as a stabbing, searing, cutting, or burning pain during vaginal penetration by their partner's penis, a pinkie, or even a tampon. Others say that a touch or tongue on their clitoris or vulva sends them into sharp, piercing, spasms of pain. Still others talk about the throbbing raw feeling that follows them for hours or days after intercourse. Many talk about the pressure to urinate that makes them feel that their bladder will explode during and after sex. There are women with irritable bowel syndrome who say that constipation can make intercourse feel like a sword is stabbing their intestines.

However, sexual pain doesn't only refer to pain during intercourse or other sexual activity, and it's not only the sexually active who suffer. Early into this project, Dr. Echenberg examined me. He said I had chronic pelvic pain (CPP), among a plethora of other conditions. I looked at him like he was from Mars. What the heck did that have to do with pain inside my vagina? I thought the pelvis was comprised of the bones that make up the cradle in which the organs sit "down there." Therefore, it seemed to me that pelvic pain must have to do with bone pain.

CHRONIC PELVIC PAIN IS THE UMBRELLA

Only after becoming educated by Dr. Echenberg and his staff did I understand that pelvic pain is the umbrella term under which all of my conditions and symptoms intersect. *Chronic pelvic pain* is the name for ongoing or intermittent pain of any or all the organs and systems between the belly button and thighs. So this included pain from conditions such as irritable bowel syndrome, bladder inflammation, lower back spasm, and, yes, the agonizing pain inside my vagina.

According to the International Pelvic Pain Society (IPPS), CPP is one of the most common medical problems affecting women today, estimated to affect 1/5 to 1/7 of American women aged 18 to 50. Shockingly, another statistic from the IPPS is that of these millions of sufferers, 61 percent have still not been diagnosed with CPP and continue spiraling downward into the abyss of despair and pain. The most important statistic for readers of this book, however, is that 80 to 90 percent of all patients with chronic pelvic pain have some type of sexual pain disorder (pain upon vaginal penetration, during sex, and/ or after sexual activity), and that is usually what finally propels them into the doctor's office.[1]

While *Secret Suffering* is a book about sex, pain, and intimacy, not a medical textbook, it's important for you to understand the causes and mechanisms of your sexual and pelvic pain. You may be surprised to learn that a lot of other disorders affecting you may be intertwined with your symptoms. Once you understand the connection between your sexual pain and other parts of your body, you'll be able to piece together the puzzle of your chronic illness and hopefully feel more confident in working with your health care provider to find relief. The information in this chapter is a good starting point.

PELVIC PAIN CAN STRIKE ANYWHERE, ANYTIME

Outside the bedroom, millions of women and young girls experience excruciating sensations in the genital area as they move through their day, causing some to leave their jobs, drop out of school, become alienated from friends and family, and lose their dreams and, sometimes, even the will to live.

Simple activities such as exercising, sitting, and wearing jeans or even underwear can trigger and aggravate the pain for some women. For others, the agony is just a constant companion.

Lori is a 23-year-old woman who has lived with pelvic pain for over 6 years. She poignantly described her feelings about this constant companion:

> There isn't anything that alienates quite like pain. It's a burning, throbbing, jabbing mess that can only truly be understood by the person experiencing it. For me, dealing with chronic pain every day is like jumping into a frigid pool.
>
> If I'm allowed to adjust to the pain, it isn't so bad. But sometimes I'm blessed with slight relief, and being plunged back into pain is miserable. I'm never given the chance to get used to the change. I'm thrust from the warm pool of summer into the icy water of winter.
>
> It's a horrible place to be, caught between hope and disappointment. It's this loss of hope when the pain returns after experiencing relief that causes me such agony. I begin to believe the brief warmth is cruelly teasing me, and part of me starts to hate the sunlight because I know every time I must return to the cold will simply be that much more unbearable. Sometimes, I'd rather just get used to the icy water.

SEX CHATTER

I spoke with many women who would never have discussed their sex life, much less their genitals, before their problems began. However, now that their lives had been taken over by this seemingly demonic force, even the most prudish among them had no compunction describing sensations in this most private part of their bodies, or graphic details of their sexual experiences. Ironically, it occurred to me that if they were describing *pleasurable* sexual feelings, *Secret Suffering* might be categorized as soft porn. But sex, anger, and frustration make strange bedfellows.

I remember the 77-year-old widow who called me crying, begging for help to find relief for vaginal burning that was driving her to suicidal despondency. Lois, another interviewee in her 50s, said, "The vaginal pain feels like somebody took pliers and grabbed hold 'down there,' twisting that whole area so it hurt beyond belief." One survey respondent described her pain as "a clenching feeling" and said, "My whole lower body tightens up. It feels like a sharp needle stabbing the right side of my clitoris."

A PICTURE IS WORTH A THOUSAND WORDS

To better understand the medical concepts presented in this chapter, it will be helpful to take a look at the pelvic area to get a clearer understanding of what's really going on down there. Figure 2.1 is a picture of the female pelvis, one that you've no doubt seen hanging in your gynecologist's examining room.

So, what's wrong with this picture? According to Dr. Echenberg, it's misleading because the image makes it look like the uterus and ovary are nearly level with the navel. But unless you're 14 to 16 weeks pregnant, this illustration is just not accurate.

Do you see the shaded, smaller structures? That's *really* the location of your uterus and ovaries. Based on this simplistic picture of the primary organs of the pelvis, when women go to the emergency room or see their doctors and point out the pain as being on either side of the lower abdomen, they are too often incorrectly told the pain is caused by their ovaries.

I remembered in my late 20s and early 30s, I had what I called a sharp, "pointy" pain in my right side when I ovulated. It scared the heck out of me, and they did an ultrasound. All they found was a tiny cyst . . . on my left side. Sometimes, I was doubled over in-between periods or had to just lie flat on the bed for a day. I was one of the so-called lucky ones. Nobody ever figured out what the problem was, so they dismissed it as ovarian pain, but they never sug-

Figure 2.1
Illustration of Commonly Displayed Female Pelvis (Courtesy of Susan Krause, CMI)

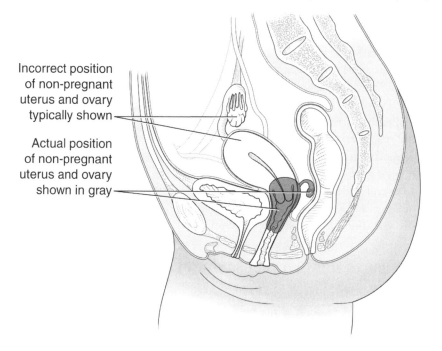

Incorrect position of non-pregnant uterus and ovary typically shown —

Actual position of non-pregnant uterus and ovary shown in gray —

gested removing my ovary. Maybe it was because I finally became disgusted with the doctors and stopped complaining about the pain to them.

Dr. Echenberg agreed. "If the pain is severe enough, an ultrasound or CT scan is performed. Many times there actually *is* a small ovarian cyst." Case solved, right? The doctors can blame the cyst for the pain (or ovulation or adhesions around the cyst) even if it hasn't ruptured or appears on the opposite side of the pain spot.

Most of the time, however, the fact is that many other issues can be triggering the pain. This is not to say that cysts are never the cause of the pain. The appearance of a cyst must be addressed and the cyst removed if needed. But further investigation is warranted if the pain persists after resolving any ovarian issues.

Unfortunately, when women do start out with this symptom and a cyst is found, what might follow can be particularly heart-wrenching for those who haven't yet had children. According to Dr. Echenberg:

> Such young women are labeled as having "recurrent cyst problems." They and their doctors believe that every time they get a pain in either lower quadrant of their abdomen that it must be their ovary.
>
> This would not be problematic in its own right, but many invasive procedures are commonly performed for these "cysts," and the patient continues to have recurrent pain. Too many times an ovary is even removed because of this sequence of events.

If the young woman continues with the same pain following removal of her gynecological parts, she is referred to another specialist. A doctor's common refrain: "There is nothing else in there that could hurt. Everything we looked at is normal." In fact, a great many things could be causing the problem, including nerves, muscles, and ligaments.

THERE'S MORE THAN MEETS THE EYE

Figure 2.1 only shows the tip of the iceberg when it comes to the complete anatomy of the pelvis. Figure 2.2 is a far more realistic version of what's actually located in the pelvic area. As you can see in Figure 2.2, a complex web of nerves, muscles, and ligaments actually make up the pelvis rather than the clear-cut, pristine image we just saw. And *all* of this stuff can trigger pelvic and sexual pain. Pretty startling contrast, don't you think?

THE PSOAS MUSCLE

In Figure 2.2, you can see a large muscle called the psoas. Like any other muscle, the psoas can go into spasm. When it does, it can feel like a charlie horse. These large muscles, located on either side of the spinal column and

Figure 2.2
Illustration of Pelvic Region Showing the Rest of the Story (Courtesy of Susan Krause, CMI)

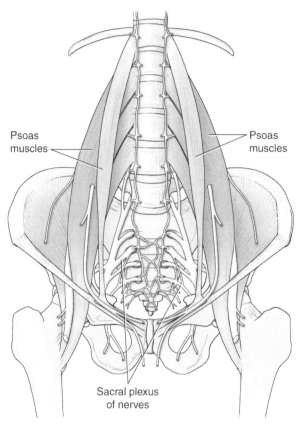

extending from the diaphragm down to the deep pelvis, are very important in stabilizing and controlling all movements involved in our torso, such as pivoting, rotating, flexing, and extending on our pelvis and lower extremities.

Consequently, when stressed or in spasm, these muscles can and do play a big part in CPP and chronic low back pain, and when in sudden spasm, they can even cause stabbing type pains going from the lower and mid-abdomen through to the back! Because so many doctors don't know about this muscle and its ability to trigger the same symptomatic pain as we've discussed, it's often overlooked as a cause of the problem.

A patient of Dr. Echenberg said, "My psoas muscle was the big trigger with me. I kept saying that my appendix felt like it was going to rupture, but it was my psoas muscle. Dr. Echenberg sent me to physical therapy, which really helped." Unfortunately, the psoas muscle looks the same on scans whether it's in normal tone or in a high state of spasm. Therefore, during an examination, a doctor should always consider the possibility that the psoas, or other muscles, are in spasm and may be causing the pain.

Valerie is a woman in great shape. A marketing director for an ad agency, she works out two hours a day. The good and bad news for women like Valerie is that they are used to "working through the pain" at the gym, which is the worst possible attitude when it comes to sexual pain.

Valerie's husband is supportive, and she says, "He's pretty laid back about everything." But when he wants sex and she tells him, "I don't want to do that because it bothers my psoas muscle," his response is, "'Well, don't you have to just keep having intercourse? When your other muscles are sore, you work them out at the gym.' We haven't had sex in more than two years because I'm afraid. Even tampons set me off. I've read on the online support groups about women who accommodate their husbands and they flare every single time."

FACTS ABOUT SEXUAL PAIN

A few of the more common conditions linked to sexual pain are endometriosis, vulvodynia, vulvar vestibulitis, and skin conditions such as lichen sclerosis. But researchers have even found a connection between sexual and pelvic pain and syndromes such as interstitial cystitis, fibromyalgia, irritable bowel syndrome, low back pain, temporomandibular joint (TMJ), and migraines. Further, doctors have found that a high proportion of women with sexual pain also experience the following symptoms:[2]

- Urinary urgency and nighttime voiding
- Constipation or diarrhea
- Vaginal or vulvar itching, burning, and sensitivity
- Lower back and/or lower abdominal pains
- Sleep problems
- Chronic fatigue

Dr. Bruce Kahn, a gynecologist at Scripps Clinic in San Diego, California, routinely screens his patients for endometriosis, interstitial cystitis, irritable bowel syndrome, fibromyalgia, migraines, and other types of headaches. He reported that half the pelvic pain patients he sees also get migraines and indicated that:

> people who have interstitial cystitis more commonly have fibromyalgia and migraines than the general public. And then there's this whole body of evidence about endometriosis' connection with interstitial cystitis: the evil twins of pelvic pain, as many of the experts call these conditions. In fact, some doctors think interstitial cystitis, endometriosis, and irritable bowel syndrome are really all the same thing.[3]

Dr. Echenberg added, "At the least, all these conditions can trigger the same pain responses."

I have migraines, fibromyalgia, irritable bowel syndrome, and interstitial cystitis. It was mind-blowing to realize that there is so much more going on in my body than meets the eye. For me, all of these seemingly unrelated illnesses converge into one big rubber band ball of pain. Like many women, it would never have occurred to me to tell my gastroenterologist or rheumatologist about my vaginal burning. Nor would it have occurred to them to ask.

ENDOMETRIOSIS AND SEXUAL PAIN

Endometriosis is a condition where the same type of tissue that exists in the uterus grows outside of it and adheres to surrounding organs, causing swelling and inflammation. Unlike the endometrial tissue in the uterus, it's not sloughed off during menstruation. These bits of tissue, called lesions, can be extremely painful but are usually not the entire cause of a patient's sexual pain.

Valerie was diagnosed with endometriosis and had two laparoscopies to remove small cysts from her ovaries. A year later, she began experiencing severe pain on her right side. Her doctor prescribed antibiotics for a bladder infection as well as treating a yeast infection.

But her symptoms didn't go away. "I continued feeling like I had a bladder infection. The doctor treated it over and over, despite finding no bacteria on cultures." After continuing on antibiotics for months, she went for an MRI and CT scan. Her OB/GYN examined her extensively and did an ultrasound. A urologist performed additional tests, but after all was said and done, the pain returned. Valerie said, "Nobody knew what was wrong. The OB/GYN thought scar tissue from the endometriosis must be causing my pain."

The relationship between endometriosis and sexual pain is becoming a somewhat controversial topic. Vast numbers of women are diagnosed with this condition and told that it is the sole cause of their discomfort. Even after treatment (with birth control pills, hormonal therapy, nonsteroidal anti-inflammatory drugs [NSAIDs], or, in extreme cases, surgery), many are left with no relief. The doctors dismiss their continuing pain as caused by residual scarring because there's no apparent organic cause for the problem.

ENDOMETRIOSIS AND INTERSTITIAL CYSTITIS

Interstitial cystitis (IC) is an inflammatory condition of the bladder wall, which is also called painful bladder syndrome (PBS/IC). It shares some of the same symptoms as a urinary tract infection, such as urgency and frequency, but there are no bacteria and it's a chronic condition. Typically, Dr. C. Lowell Parsons, urologist and professor of surgery at the University of

California at San Diego, won't point to endometriosis as the cause of sexual/pelvic pain. In his opinion, "a patient may have some endometriosis, but it has nothing to do with the patient's pelvic pain." Dr. Kahn agreed, adding, "The symptoms of endometriosis and PBS/IC are basically identical."

Some doctors think interstitial cystitis is the primary culprit in triggering sexual pain symptoms. According to Dr. Parsons, if you have pain or symptoms that are associated with sex, there's over an 80 percent chance it's coming from your bladder.[4] This pervasive condition is often missed because doctors don't screen for IC, and therefore, patients are mistakenly diagnosed with urinary tract infections, despite negative cultures. Furthermore, many women have symptoms of IC but never tell their doctors; they've spent so many years with urinary frequency and urgency that they assume it's normal. It's a shame, because there are tools and treatments if only doctors would use them.

Dr. Parsons talked about how doctors dealt with IC patients in 1980, when little was known about the condition. He said that patients came into the doctor's office with severe symptoms and were usually older by the time they were diagnosed. According to Dr. Parsons,

> No one asked that 55-year-old what she was like when she was 25. She probably had classic symptoms even then, including sexual pain, but they weren't continuous over the years. She may have had almost no symptoms for a long period, but no one picked up on the fact that the disease has a lengthy, insidious progression. In fact, one out of four women, even at age 23, has this sort of chronic, active intermittent symptomatology.[5]

It's believed that up to 25 percent of all American women suffer from IC during their reproductive years.[6] Dr. Parsons said, "These data suggest the estimate of IC prevalence in the US should be vastly increased from approximately 1.5 million to perhaps 25–30 million women, and that IC is highly prevalent in young women."[7]

What a survey respondent wrote reflects Dr. Parsons' experience:

> I am 44 years old and developed signs of IC six months into a sexual relationship with my now estranged husband. I had other long-term sexual relationships but they never caused this type of pain. It took over four years to be diagnosed with IC and it eventually tore our relationship apart.
>
> As a child, I was constantly diagnosed with kidney infections and urinary tract infections (UTIs). I had horrible urethral dilations performed on me when I was three and four. The symptoms went away in my teens and early twenties. But once I was with my husband, the IC symptoms came back in full force.

Apparently, for many medical professionals, little has changed in all these years, which means that many thousands, if not millions, of women haven't reaped the benefit of early diagnosis and treatment.

JENNIFER, THE MODEL PATIENT

Jennifer, who is now 25, had been to the emergency room innumerable times since she was 15 for pain on her left side, which was variously diagnosed as mittelschmerz (ovulatory pain) or caused by burst cysts. Over subsequent years, she saw more than six OB/GYN doctors and took numerous types of birth control pills to control painful periods and times in-between, but they never worked. As for the attitude of those doctors, she said, "They basically told me to 'push the pain under the carpet' and pull myself up by my boot-straps. They said that I was just 'doing this' for attention."

Because she needed to find some reason for what she went through every month, she convinced herself that she could "chalk up the pain to endometrio-sis" since her mother had the condition. Jennifer explained:

> The idea of endometriosis was the one thing I could hold on to and say, "This is why I feel the way I do." I finally had laparoscopic surgery last year, only to find out I don't have endometriosis. This came as a shock to everyone, including the doctor who performed the surgery. I was crestfallen and in disbelief. I thought I'd never find a way to feel better, and would have to live with this pain forever.

Jennifer's partner, Lisa, observed how difficult it is to watch someone you love suffer through a seemingly unending cycle of pain. She remembered Jennifer's hopes crumbling after finding out that her pain wasn't caused by endometriosis. On the other hand, Lisa "couldn't be more grateful" for the miraculous change of fortune that occurred because Jennifer's doctors were out of ideas. Six months after the procedure, she was referred to Dr. Echenberg. Jennifer described their first meeting:

> I had a two-hour consultation with an exam. Dr. Echenberg pointed out that what I thought were the normal aches and pains other women felt actually stemmed from chronic pelvic pain syndrome. My diagnoses were vulvodynia, interstitial cystitis, irritable bowel syndrome, and pelvic floor dysfunction.

She was prescribed physical therapy to work on strengthening the muscles in and around the pelvic area that were constantly in spasm. She received Lupron shots once a month to give her body a break from menstrual pain so she could focus on other aspects of her condition.

Jennifer received bladder instillations once a week, changed her diet, and took medication to quiet inflamed nerves. It took roughly two months for the IC urinary symptoms to be controlled, which reduced her urgency and frequency to urinate. She has also been getting pudendal nerve shots, which she said hurt a great deal. However, she noted, "The way I see it, for a few minutes of pain I can get relief for a full week. I know eventually the relief will last longer and longer, so to me, it's worth it."

Jennifer's positive experience with Dr. Echenberg has been replicated by patients all over the world who have found doctors like him and those interviewed for *Secret Suffering*. This positive phenomenon is due to the growing number of doctors who have found the desire and willingness to learn about pelvic pain and walk the long road with their patients to help them find relief. Obviously, Jennifer's treatment plan is unique to her, and not all of these excellent physicians treat pelvic and sexual pain the same way. But they all share the same passion and dedication to validating their patients' experiences and helping them recover their lives.

Jennifer said, "At Dr. Echenberg's office, I didn't feel like I was just another numbered patient that needed to be seen and checked out quickly, or that I was in some sort of OB/GYN factory. Finally, I began to believe that life without excessively high levels of daily pain might be possible. That's when I knew I could have a love life again with my partner."

DISCOMFORT VERSUS PAIN

I asked Lisa Fournace, a nurse practitioner at Heritage Women's Center in Nashville, Tennessee, what percentage of her patients have sexual pain. She said, "When most of my patients come to me, their sexual pain is a big component of what's going on." However, she told me that some of her patients have no clue they're experiencing sexual pain along with their other conditions:

> For instance, if they have interstitial cystitis and I touch their bladders, they'll say, "Oh that's uncomfortable" so I ask if they experience that sensation with intercourse. When they respond affirmatively, I say, "Don't you count that as pain?"
>
> Only then do they put it together. Finally, they say, "Actually yes, but I never associated it with sex." Some women think this is a normal sensation and call it "discomfort." They usually say "it doesn't feel good "or "I feel too tight and he's pushing too hard" or "it hurts." They reserve the word *pain* to describe a far more severe feeling.

So I have concluded that discomfort and pain are the same thing. In fact, I see chronic sexual pain as a devious opponent, a silent enemy that can cover its victim with a veil of denial. Itching is one powerful example of a sensation that is included in the pain category but wouldn't be described as such by most women, including myself. Then I remembered having yeast infections and wanting to stick a loofah in there and scratch it raw. As one survey respondent said, "I experience intense itching on my vulva like I've never known before! Nothing helps! This is such an awful, hopeless feeling!" If that isn't pain, I don't know what is.

ADJUSTING TO FUNCTION

You've definitely crossed the threshold of discomfort into pain if you have to change your life to accommodate it, and the degree to which you have to alter your daily activities to experience any relief corresponds to the severity of the pain. The consequences of those changes range from slight to profoundly heartbreaking.

For instance, if you know that pushing a vacuum cleaner around hurts your lower back, you may have extremely dirty carpets. If the slight pressure of underwear on your genitals makes you want to climb the walls, you might have to cut holes in them or do without them altogether. If you are a teacher and standing all day makes you feel as if your bottom is literally falling out because of extreme pressure, you may need to leave a career you love. Finally, if you stop all sexual activity with your partner because you cannot walk for hours afterwards because your vagina is throbbing with a ripping pain, your relationship may not be able to survive.

LIVING WITH CPP: SUSAN'S JOURNAL

Today, while reading through transcripts of the interviews for *Secret Suffering*, I started to cry. I'm crying because I hurt. I have an ache—actually many of them—but the one that presides today is the pressure hose of a bladder, this feeling that I have to go, really have to go . . . all the time. It's a chronic, low-grade pressure, a "toothache" down there, as one of the survey respondents called it. I go to the bathroom and pee, a hot strong stream. I think I'm done, but I sit there for another 10 seconds and out pours more. Done. But I still feel like I have to go. It's a haunting feeling, not really a pain. Just a constant companion.

Then there's the agonizing feeling of being scraped with the sharp edge of a knife during intercourse. It's been awhile since I've been in remission from pain so that intercourse felt bearable. Even when I want sex, which is rarely, being touched *anywhere* in my genital region often feels excruciating.

In the process of writing this book, I have occasionally stepped back from the project and looked at those with the courage to write and talk to me. It seems as if they are somehow different from me. They really have it rough.

Then I reviewed my situation. I have fibromyalgia, pelvic floor dysfunction, vulvodynia, vestibulitis, and more. *I am these women.* In fact, I'm a difficult case because I can find no doctors in Florida who want to deal with the complexities of chronic pelvic pain, no doctors who are willing to treat the sum of the parts, and no doctors who want to become educated about CPP. Plus, I have multiple chemical sensitivities that prevent me from taking many of the medications that may help.

Because of this, what I have learned to do is sublimate my pain. No, not the pain itself, but the *impact* of the pain. Dr. Echenberg calls it acclimating to higher and higher levels of discomfort. Once in a while, however, a flare-up reminds me that I have these conditions, and I complain about my aching joints, aching vagina, and aching head. Plus, the flames of my "burning bush," to be rather crass, have begun to intensify outside the bedroom lately, even when sitting in my computer chair, wearing jeans, and just living my life. My husband looks at me, sees someone who appears to be healthy, and simply says, with a click of the tongue, "Oh, you're always whining about your health."

I'm only 53. Usually I say, "Ugh, I'm already 53." But in this case, my age desperately prompts me to want to feel better because I have a chance at a few more decades on this earth. I'm sure I'll have another remission from all of this and feel much better (I hope), but the truth for me is, I may feel better once in awhile, but I'll probably never get well.

We live in a world where people expect a magic pill to fix their ills. Accepting that pelvic and sexual pain may be a chronic illness is a difficult "pill" for women to swallow. When women combine this "pill" with the unfortunate message the media pounds into our heads—that if we aren't having hot, steamy sex, there's something wrong with us—it's easy to become demoralized.

Therefore, sometimes, like the day described here, I just cry and sink into the pain and self-pity. I allow it to blanket me, and I feel helpless and demoralized. On other days, I just ignore it and move on.

It's important to remember that everyone has *something* to deal with. No one escapes life unscathed. I am comforted by the philosophy that we're here on earth to overcome obstacles, that no one has a free ride. Certainly, it's true that many have it much worse and many have it much better. Jane, one of the *Secret Suffering* interviewees, has tried to alter her perception of the illness. She said, "I guess my belief is that I have been dealt a bad card and this card is probably going to stay with me for the rest of my life."

I'm reminded of Randy Pausch, the late Carnegie-Mellon professor and author of *The Last Lecture*. He died in 2008 of pancreatic cancer, leaving behind a wife and three small children. His take on that card deck is, "We cannot change the cards we are dealt, just how we play the hand."[8]

I listened to an online recording of the "last lecture" he gave at Carnegie-Mellon University many months before he died. In his talk, he celebrated his life and accepted the inevitable death that was inching ever closer, and I learned something important about how to handle my own illness. Randy Pausch didn't let his disease control his attitude. It may have controlled his destiny, but not his ability to face his fate head on with humor, courage, and the determination to do all he could to savor the time he had left on this earth.

PUTTING LIFE IN PERSPECTIVE

There is an expression that says, "Pain is what I walk through; misery is what I sit in." For some women, it helps to remember that CPP will not be the only challenge they face. Nor may it be the worst.

Fifty-four-year-old Ellen and her husband, married for decades, have sexual activity once a week or less due to the pain of interstitial cystitis and vulvar vestibulitis. She recalled other times over the long span of their marriage that they were unable to have sex at all, such as when her husband had a frozen shoulder or she had surgery for another condition. She offered ways relationships can weather such difficulties:

> Couples should consider the crises they have already dealt with. If this is the first crisis, would they consider it the equivalent of a broken fingernail or a broken arm?
>
> Well, the broken fingernail is nothing and the broken arm is a bigger deal. Your perspective as to what you want, what you need, and what you expect depends on your life experiences and background.
>
> I go for swimming rehabilitation. Many others who are there are in such bad shape that I conclude my problem isn't all that big. So I keep my mouth shut and just deal with what I've been given for that day.

Ellen's attitude of gratitude and acceptance of what life puts in front of her reminds me of the "Serenity Prayer" (whose origin is unknown but cherished by millions of recovering alcoholics and addicts around the world):

> God grant us the serenity to accept the things we cannot change, courage to change the things we can, and wisdom to know the difference.

To that, I'd like to add another prayer, one passed on to me decades ago by a woman who suffered from many painful, chronic physical conditions. She told me that praying to feel better usually leads to frustration. Instead, she suggested, "Help me to bear the discomfort until comfort comes."

Ain't that the truth? For CPP patients, comfort may never come, or it may come in dribs and drabs, but the message for me in both of those prayers is that intestinal fortitude (no pun intended) and hope go hand in hand.

Whether comfort arrives or not isn't in my hands. All I can do is continue trying to get better and accept my condition on days when nothing helps at all. My mantra is to keep moving forward until you hit a brick wall, and then, just turn and keep moving in another direction.

Chapter Three

CHRISTIN VEASLEY: PERSONAL PAIN AND PROFESSIONAL PASSION

Christin Veasley (Chris) is the associate executive director of the National Vulvodynia Association (NVA). In addition, she is one of the millions of women who have suffered with chronic sexual/pelvic pain. As a courageous and outspoken advocate for women with vulvodynia, Chris was willing to share her personal story as well as her insights on the subject of sexual pain.

SUFFERING ACUTE TRAUMA AND PELVIC PAIN

At the age of 15, Chris was hit by a car while riding her bicycle. She suffered massive internal damage and broken bones. The doctors weren't sure she would survive the accident, and she was kept in the hospital for a month. Over the next year, she experienced the severe pain of acute trauma as she went through rehabilitation to learn to walk again. Since then, she's suffered with chronic neck and back pain as a result of the accident.

In 1993, when she was 18, Chris began experiencing symptoms of vulvodynia and was eventually diagnosed with vulvar vestibulitis. When asked about how the neck/back pain compare with her pelvic pain, she said:

> None of the pain I experienced as a result of my accident compares with living with chronic genital pain. I say that because of the unrelenting nature of the pain and because of the stigma associated with it. It's not something that you feel you can easily share with people.

Disclosing a headache or back pain to someone is not the same as talking to them about your genital pain. It's very difficult and not something that people can easily understand or to which they can relate.

There's something to be said for having a community of people around you when you're suffering from any kind of illness. When that doesn't exist because you can't openly share what's going on with you, it's very isolating.

Chris described her first experiences with the nurse practitioner she saw:

I kept going back every two weeks, and she kept saying, "I don't know what this is." After a few months, she diagnosed my condition as vulvar vestibulitis syndrome, but proceeded to tell me, incorrectly I later learned, that there weren't really any treatments for it. The final straw was the day I was in the middle of a physics exam and I couldn't sit or concentrate because of the severity of the pain.

I thought, "It can't be possible that women are walking around like this, with this burning, where they can't sit, can't wear pants."

I couldn't even finish my exam. I got up halfway through and turned it in. I drove to her office at five o'clock at night and sat crying in her waiting room.

The receptionist said, "You don't have an appointment," and I said, "I know I don't, but I'm in such pain and can't go another day like this." The nurse practitioner finally saw me and after a brief conversation handed me what turned out to be a life-saving piece of paper: a photocopied brochure from the newly formed National Vulvodynia Association. She told me that maybe they could help me.

Chris took matters into her own hands by educating herself about her condition and researching local doctors. As the months passed, the pain changed from "only on touch" to all the time. Six months after her diagnosis, she found a local obstetrician-gynecologist at the University of Wisconsin Hospital who was knowledgeable and empathic. Over the next seven years, she religiously tried almost every treatment available for vulvodynia with only minor improvement. A combination of treatments helped to alleviate the 24/7 pain she experienced, but she was still left with severe vestibular pain with touch or vaginal penetration.

WHEN A VESTIBULECTOMY WORKS

In 2000, Chris decided to have surgery for the vestibulitis. She found a knowledgeable gynecologist (now a chronic pelvic pain specialist) who was willing to partner with her, as opposed to the traditional omnipotent management style of many physicians. She said, "At that point, I had tried every treatment available, other than interferon injections and surgery. I decided to proceed with my doctor's recommendation. I trusted his knowledge and skill. Women ask me this question all the time: What's most important to consider when selecting a doctor? Certainly, you need somebody who is knowledgeable, but his/her willingness to partner with you is also very important."

The surgery was a success. She had a four- to six-week recovery period, during which she and her husband started seeing a sex therapist. She was taught to use dilators to help relax her muscles and was able to have intercourse for the first time in seven years. Within three months of the surgery, Chris was pregnant, and to this day, the vestibulitis hasn't returned.

Chris admits that the surgery is not for everyone: "Research indicates that surgery seems to be most effective for a select group of women who have vestibular pain with touch or pressure *only* and don't suffer with several concomitant conditions. It is never recommended for the treatment of generalized vulvodynia."

I related to what she was saying. My own gynecologist advised me to have a vestibulectomy. However, I have a lot of those concomitant conditions, such as pudendal neuralgia, pelvic floor dysfunction, vulvodynia, fibromyalgia, and irritable bowel syndrome. The tip-off that this wasn't a good option for me was the fact that during physical therapy I wasn't able to tell the difference between the pain when the physical therapist pressed on the vestibule at the opening of my vagina and when she massaged a tight internal trigger point. They felt one and the same. I also realized I might not want to go this route when my doctor warned that the vestibulitis might return after the surgery. There was no question that the surgery *might* remove one pain trigger, but it would leave a boatload of others. Unfortunately, there's no magic wand or surgery to sweep away the problems of multisymptom patients like myself.

Chris added that a small number of research studies have started to provide preliminary data as to which factors may be associated with a successful surgical outcome, but much more research is needed.

HOW WOMEN HANDLE RELATIONSHIPS

Chris said that young women like herself often have a slew of issues to work through, whether they have a partner or not. She listed a number of questions women ask that can create additional turmoil as they try to heal:

> Will I ever find a partner who can deal with this?
> Will I ever be able to get pregnant?
> Am I going to have to take these medications for the rest of my life?

Single women with sexual pain who may or may not be dating have their own special set of problems. For instance, when do you disclose your condition to someone you're dating? Even worse, how on earth can you explain it and expect your partner to stick around?

Chris said that some women don't want to deal with it at all. They just don't date. Many are filled with fear and anxiety at the prospect of rejection.

Women who have developed the condition after years in a relationship find that it completely changes the nature of that relationship. Chris said, "We've heard from many women whose marriages have dissolved over this. They find that the change in intimacy level between them is very difficult to deal with."

Another major relationship concern she's heard is the difficulty of convincing your partner that you are, indeed, ill after seeing doctor after doctor who may dismiss your problems out of hand and say it's all in your head. She said, "The partner may start saying, 'Well, the doctor said everything is fine. There can't be anything wrong with you.' So, in some cases, women have told us that in addition to their doctor not believing them, now their significant other doesn't believe them either."

Chris said that knowledgeable physicians encourage couples to continue being intimate in ways that don't hurt; otherwise, there is a cycle of rejection, anxiety, and fear associated with any kind of sexual relationship or activity that can spill over after the woman feels better. But, according to Chris, "Whether this works depends upon the willingness of both partners to explore other intimacy options. It takes a lot of effort, but it is attainable."

Chris has worked with a vast number of women with vulvodynia, first as a support group leader and now as the Associate Director of the NVA. She thinks that it's very important for women who recover to give others hope by sharing their success stories. She said, "Support, whether it be in the form of group meetings or online chats, is very important. But, often times, there can be a misguided perception that no one ever gets better and that can be very dangerous to a woman who is newly diagnosed. Women do get better."

BE YOUR OWN ADVOCATE FOR YOUR HEALTH

The NVA maintains a list of providers for patient referral. Chris told me that in the mid-1990s, the NVA started with 50 providers. Today, there are about 500. But even with the increase in health care professionals who have some knowledge about vulvodynia and related disorders, Chris said that women must continue to be their own advocate:

> I recently read an article about five mistakes women routinely make when visiting their doctors. The best advice from the article was for women to trust their own instincts. Too many of us accept what health care providers say without question, even when we're not convinced that they are knowledgeable.
>
> I've heard time and time again about cancers that were undiagnosed in women. They're told, "Nothing is wrong with you" or "you're 28 years old" or "you're 35 years old" and it couldn't possibly be cancer ... but they were wrong. The women inevitably say, "I just knew something wasn't right," but they didn't pursue it because "the doctor said I was fine."

Chris said it's difficult to push for awareness on these issues when she and others from the NVA go to Capitol Hill or talk to the National Institute of Health (NIH) and media. "First," she said, "chronic pain conditions aren't seen as life threatening and they're not communicable, so they're given lower priority." What they clearly don't understand is that *living* with these conditions every day often makes life unbearable.

More young patients contact the NVA now, highlighting the fact that the first symptoms may present at an earlier age than previously thought. Internet savvy youth may find it easier to research their symptoms and ask for help. Chris added, "It's a different mentality now. My mother grew up in a time when you didn't question the doctor—ever! I have a completely different perception of how the patient/provider relationship should function. I look at it as a team, a relationship between the two (or more) of us."

As we wrapped up our interview, Chris again stressed that women must not give up hope. She said, "My best advice to women is to trust your own instinct, educate yourself, and become your own advocate. There are so many more resources available to women now than when I suffered. Don't give up hope. You can get better!"

Chapter Four

UNDERSTANDING CHRONIC PAIN AND YOUR NERVOUS SYSTEM

My feet hurt all the time because, when I walk, I tend to keep my crotch area farther apart than a normal person would, so it won't cause further irritation. This one square inch of my body needs to go somewhere else.

—Lauren (interviewee)

My husband and I would be sitting at home and I'd have to go every 20 minutes. I've had this pattern since I was in college. My friends joked about "Jane and her tiny little bladder."

—Jane (interviewee)

For a long time, wearing anything other than loose clothing aggravated the pain. In fact, if I walked, sat, climbed, or bent up and down, the pain worsened. Nothing other than lying flat gave me relief.

—Lois (interviewee)

For years, I've had to be careful in my clothing selection, cautious in my food choices, conscious where I sit (hard chairs hurt), diligent in finding restrooms. Worst of all, I often have to choose between pushing away a sexual encounter and disappointing my partner, or suffering through it.

—Susan (author)

Patients and their health care providers deal with two kinds of pain: acute and chronic. In explaining the difference between acute and chronic pelvic/sexual pain, Dr. Bruce Kahn, a gynecologist at Scripps Clinic in San Diego, California, said, "Women with acute pain come in with, for instance, an ovarian cyst, a bladder infection, appendicitis, and so on. They get treated for the condition and go on with their lives. Chronic pain is very different. It can affect whether and how you can work, and how you function with family and friends." The latter requires dealing with a syndrome for the rest of your life—one that affects those around you and your whole lifestyle.

Physicians have been primarily trained to deal with all pain as acute pain. Traditionally, it's been the doctor's job to find out what specific tissue damage is causing the pain and fix it. Acute pain is a necessary warning system throughout our bodies. Our brain needs to know if we have stepped on a sharp nail, broken our ankle, or if we're having a heart attack so that we can react to protect ourselves from further injury or even death.

In contrast to acute pain, chronic pain serves no basic survival function; in fact, it serves no helpful function at all. According to the International Pelvic Pain Society (IPPS), "Although acute pain may indicate specific active injury to some part of the body, chronic pain is very different. Often in chronic pelvic pain, the initial physical problem has lessened or even disappeared, but the pain continues because of changes in the nervous system, muscles, or other tissues."

YOU'RE *NOT* CRAZY, BUT THE PROBLEM *IS* IN YOUR HEAD

Neuroscientist and pelvic pain researcher Dr. Karen Berkley has spent her career studying pain in general, and the last 10 to 15 years focused on the interrelationship of the pelvic organs and central nervous system. She said:

> When you get told that pain is all in your head, you get angry, right? But it's *always* in your head, no matter what. You stub your toe—it's in your head . . . because the stimulus is not the perception.
>
> You stub your toe, that's a *stimulus*, but that, in and of itself is not *pain*. Pain is what your nervous system makes of the information about that stubbed toe, in relationship to what is going on around you at the time. So, on some occasions the stubbed toe may not even hurt in the moment because you're busy saving somebody from being hit by a car, for instance.
>
> In other words, the information is taken on-board by the nervous system but it's not always translated into pain because some other stimuli take precedence, such as seeing a child running into the street in front of a car or hearing an alarm go off telling you to "evacuate the building."[1]

Dr. Echenberg explained that even acute pain from severe injury doesn't always get to the brain for the individual to react protectively. Ironically, if something more crucial is happening to the person in that moment, the pain may be gated (or blocked) from getting to the brain temporarily until the crisis is over. Our nervous system recognizes and prioritizes what's most important at any given moment, for instance, either the stubbed toe or saving the child. It's not a matter of denying the pain or that the nervous system is turning off the pain, but as Dr. Berkley said, "It's changing the interpretation of all the stimuli going on at that moment, in the context of what's been learned about living over a lifetime."

Let's take another example. It's three o'clock in the morning and you hear a loud thumping at your front door. You stub that darned toe again getting out of bed. Where will you place your focus? Dr. Berkley said, "The nervous system automatically arranges priorities. Do you need to take care of your toe or do you need to take care of your entire body by going into a closet and finding something with which to protect yourself from possible greater danger?"

Based on my experience, I'd automatically head to the closet with nary a thought about that little digit, unless, of course, I realized that a broken tree branch had knocked into the door, in which case I'd just be really annoyed. Then I'd be hopping on one foot to the refrigerator to get an ice pack for my now-throbbing toe.

YOUR NERVOUS SYSTEM HAS A GREAT MEMORY

According to Drs. Berkley and Echenberg, the nervous system has cumulatively stored memories of traumatic events throughout one's life, such as physical and/or emotional injuries, abuse, surgeries, intensive sports activities, and so forth. These are all part of an individual's past history and provide a guidebook to the nervous system as to how to interpret events that are happening right now. Our nervous system uses this information to not only determine *whether* you feel pain, but how, when, and where the pain shows up based on what is going on in the body at the time. "The problem is that for some people, these accumulated traumas and experiences may result in a condition called 'central sensitization,' which means the central nervous system [CNS, the brain and spinal cord] sends out pain signals in reaction to even small amounts of stimuli," said Dr. Echenberg.

Dr. Echenberg explains to each of his new patients that pain processing can play amazing tricks on the suffering individual. For example, *phantom limb pain* is a phenomenon that sometimes occurs following amputation of limbs (often after serious trauma such as war or crush injuries). The person may experience the "worst pain ever" in the amputated arm or leg, even though the limb is no longer there. In these cases, the brain is being fed old information from the region in the spinal cord where it has remained stored since the original injury. Similarly, some women continue to feel uterine and ovarian pain, even following complete removal of these organs.

Noted Dr. Kahn, "Visceral nerves (the nerves that go to your guts) down in that part of the body are hypersensitive, so something has made them not function properly. Think of it as a nerve dysfunction." His question is not whether the patient really feels the pain, he knows they do, but how to get these nerves that are sending the pain signals to calm down.

AND THE DIAGNOSIS IS . . . PAIN!

Research over the past decade has proven that traditional gynecologic diagnoses for chronic pelvic pain (CPP), such as adhesions, ovarian cysts, and endometriosis, may play a role in triggering pain during sex or pain in the genital area, but most often, they are just one small component of a far more complex disorder.[2]

Dr. Fred Howard, MS, MD, FACOG, Chairman of the Board of the International Pelvic Pain Society, Associate Chair, and Professor of Obstetrics and Gynecology at the University of Rochester Medical Center in Rochester, New York, wrote in the Foreword of his textbook *Pelvic Pain: Diagnosis and Management,* "After six months of pelvic pain, the pain itself can become an illness, rather than a symptomatic manifestation of some other disease."[3] Therefore, lingering (or chronic) pain becomes the diagnosis, invisible to our tests and our observation, but absolutely real, in neurochemical terms, absolutely experienced by the patient, and coming from pain generated within the nervous system itself.

THE ESCALATING CYCLE OF PAIN

How does the nervous system policing your sensations relate to sexual pain? Remember that every physical or emotional pain event experienced in life gets stored into memory in the central nervous system. Even minor levels of injury creep in below the level of conscious awareness and may finally spill over the edge of tolerance that a particular individual has developed over time. As Dr. Nel Gerig, urologist, said, the nervous system can detour traffic, sending it to a new destination. "All of these events add up, so their cumulative effect can be under the radar for decades. It sleeps below the level of our consciousness until some event, such as childbirth, pelvic surgery, or new physical or emotional trauma triggers it over the threshold *into* our consciousness. That's when we finally feel it," explained Dr. Gerig.

As an example, Dr. Echenberg cites a growing recognition among doctors specializing in pelvic and sexual pain that young women with CPP are often involved in sports such as gymnastics, dance, contact sports, track and field, and so on. Injuries sustained during these activities may appear to have left the girls unaffected but show up later when they display severe symptoms, as he explained, "This cumulative imprinting of pain neurochemistry in the central nervous system when these girls are young can turn into a chronic regional pain syndrome such as migraine, fibromyalgia, chronic fatigue, and chronic pelvic pain years after any sports injuries they may have sustained."

THE ENDLESS CYCLE OF SEXUAL PAIN

People can enter the cycle of chronic sexual pain from the bladder, lower bowel, reproductive organs, or after having multiple pelvic traumas, whether surgical, accidental, athletic, or all of the above. Dr. Echenberg reiterated that as any chronic pain syndrome progresses, it takes less and less stimuli to feel the same symptoms, and you may experience the pain in unrelated parts of your body. Here's how Dr. Gerig described it: "When the nerves get revved up, the nerve message pathways get screwed up, so neural pathways create their own 'on-ramps, mergers, exits, and detours.' Messages go not only from the bladder to the brain but they start to go back out to the pelvis and when they're there, they don't always go home. Sometimes they visit the neighbors."

Dr. Echenberg calls this neurologic "cross-talk" between the organs. For instance, you might have a bowel movement that makes you feel a burning sensation when you pee. Or your bladder is in spasm and your vagina starts to burn. You start feeling the labial, vulvar burning pain and then get a muscle spasm in your back and your joints inflame. You could also have a musculoskeletal issue, such as scoliosis, slipped disc, back injury, or past pelvic fracture that eventually translates into stabbing pains throughout your vulva.

This cross-talk from your bladder, lower bowel, or female organs, which can cause severe vulvar or vaginal pain, is similar to why people feel pain in their jaw and down their left arm while having a heart attack. In this case, the heart is the damaged visceral organ, but the jaw and arm become the locations of pain perceived by the victim of a coronary occlusion (heart attack).

In another example, say you fell on your butt. You were badly bruised and it hurt. That's acute pain. After awhile, the pain goes away, but the memory of the trauma to your butt gets imprinted on your nervous system, which can later send ongoing pain signals to another part of your body (usually in the same basic region). So your butt feels fine, but you might begin to experience persistent vaginal burning.

To sum it up, the entire horrid scope of CPP and sexual pain is like a row of falling dominos. Just flick one little black rectangle and each downed piece causes the next to react until the walls of Jericho come tumbling down.

THE PUDENDAL NERVE

In Figure 4.1 you can see the pudendal nerve, which is a big trigger for many types of pelvic pain. This illustration may seem a bit complex, but trust me, you *want* to know more about the pudendal nerve because it is the source of much of our sexual pain.

Figure 4.1
The Pudendal Nerve (Courtesy of Susan Krause, CMI)

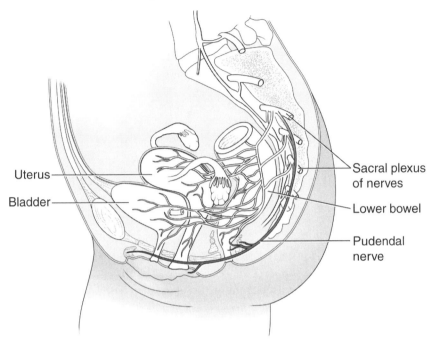

Uterus

Bladder

Sacral plexus
of nerves

Lower bowel

Pudendal
nerve

Here's how it works: The nerves of the basic organs of the pelvis (for instance, the urinary bladder) transmit pain signals into the central nervous system. Nerves from the lower portion of your back, just above your butt (the second, third, and fourth sacral nerves) funnel into the pudendal nerve. The pudendal nerve winds its way around both sides of your pelvis, through the muscles in your butt and deep into the internal pelvic muscles and ligaments, finally passing through an area very near to the hipbone called Alcock's canal. From there, the nerves on each side branch out into many smaller nerves that stimulate (make that irritate!) the entire saddle area of your bottom and connect to the entire vulvar area.

In Figure 4.2 you are looking straight into the pelvis and genital area from below. You can see the increased number of branches from the pudendal nerve, which connect directly with the sexual organs and tissues, such as the clitoris, labia, entire vulva, anus, and perineum (tissue between the vaginal opening and anus).

PELVIC FLOOR DYSFUNCTION

When pelvic pain becomes chronic, there's a corresponding spasm or contraction of the surrounding pelvic floor and pelvic side wall muscles and often a weakening of the lower abdominal wall muscles. This weakness makes the

Figure 4.2
The Pudendal Nerve: A Different View (Courtesy of Susan Krause, CMI)

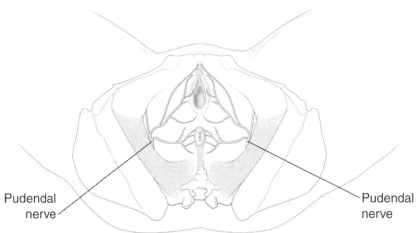

Pudendal
nerve

Pudendal
nerve

lower abdomen bulge, often causing bloating and core muscles to tighten and splint (work harder to support) the pelvis because of the continued pain, essentially trying to protect itself from further damage (clenching or splinting).

This condition is called *pelvic floor dysfunction* or *high tone pelvic floor myofascial pain*. It is almost universally found in women with chronic pelvic pain. Eventually, it becomes a vicious cycle where the nerves are firing off through the pudendals because of previous injuries, surgeries, pelvic organ dysfunctions, and sometimes emotional pain imprinting, and the muscles respond by contracting throughout the pelvis.

In Dr. Echenberg's Words

This concept (pelvic floor dysfunction or high tone pelvic floor myofascial pain) is easily understood by our patients, says Dr. Echenberg, because we describe the analogy of a shoulder or knee injury causing spasm and splinting of the surrounding muscles while the injured area recovers, following which physical therapy would be utilized for exercise and range of motion to avoid stiffness and further pain.

Unfortunately, so many people forget that there are numerous muscles in the pelvic core and that those muscles and their surrounding ligaments can also go into spasm with CPP. It would actually take a total body cast to immobilize the entire pelvis, which of course is not practical (except if the pelvis is actually fractured). No wonder then that physical therapy for the pelvic floor and low back would be needed to re-educate those muscles after being in spasm for so long (just like the need to go through rehab following other bodily injuries).

One of the things that we always check for at the first visit with our patients is the sensitivity of the pudendal nerves on both sides. This is easily done by pressing one finger of my examining hand into the area on each side of the pelvis near the bony prominence that we all sit on. This spot is not supposed to be tender or uncomfortable. A significant portion of our new patients do have some degree of tenderness on one side or both sides, precisely where the pudendal nerve exits from its tiny canal and branches out into the entire vulvar region.

We commonly find this tenderness in those patients with various combinations of diagnoses such as vulvodynia, interstitial cystitis, irritable bowel syndrome, and pelvic floor dysfunction. We also show them with a one finger exam carefully placed into the vagina that the pelvic floor and side wall muscles are not only in spasm but are very tender as well (high tone pelvic floor dysfunction). We will then gently touch the vaginal opening with a Q-tip while showing them with a mirror that the Q-tip is causing them to feel like it is a needle or a knife or a piece of sandpaper (vulvar vestibulitis).

We also carefully push on the base of the bladder in the upper part of the vagina and, surprisingly to our patients, they say that that discomfort on the bladder is often precisely the pain they have experienced for years with deep vaginal intercourse. This is the condition called interstitial cystitis (IC). Obviously, not every patient has all of these findings, but you'd be surprised at how many do.

THE ROLE OF SEX HORMONES IN PELVIC PAIN

While working as a researcher with Vernon and Wilson, who were studying fertility and endometriosis using laboratory animals developed as living models, Dr. Berkley wondered if these animals experienced vaginal pain. She said, "I knew that one of the symptoms of endometriosis in women is vaginal hyperalgesia, a very sensitive vaginal canal, which clinically may also result in dyspareunia, painful vaginal penetration, or coital sexual pain. But it's much more than that. It's not a sexual dysfunction. It's a true pain disorder."

And indeed, they did discover genital pain in the lab animals, which was the springboard for Dr. Berkley's ongoing research into "the kind of information that was being transmitted via those nerves connecting the pelvic organs to the central nervous system, and its consequences."

This was the beginning of a journey that led Dr. Berkley to attempt to improve our understanding of how the nervous system can evoke an experience of pain in a part of the body unrelated to where the initial problem occurred, as well as to the role sex hormones might play in these situations for women.

Dr. Berkley's research, for instance, has shown that hormonal changes in the menstrual cycle have a direct relationship with a network of nerves that can develop within endometriosis lesions in the pelvis. This new type of nerve growth can even cause new inflammation in the vicinity of the lesions (called neurogenic inflammation). Her work also showed that this inflammatory reaction could be significantly influenced by the sex hormones in women, especially estrogen.

In Dr. Echenberg's Words

Neurogenic inflammation is a fairly new concept in the research world of chronic pain. Pain transmission through the nerves appears to cause an actual inflammatory response at those parts of the body to which those nerves are connected. Therefore, pain itself, which may be generating from the central nervous system, seems to reach out through the peripheral nerves (nerves that run from your spinal cord to all other parts of your body).

This causes the body to have a protective response (inflammation), just as when the body responds to protect us against the invasion of pathogenic bacteria or fungal organisms. It is important to note that this phenomenon may explain why so many young women are treated over and over for vaginal yeast infections when the diagnosis is often vestibulitis. Often, the nerves to the vaginal opening become highly irritated in association with long-standing interstitial cystitis, irritable bowel, painful periods, and so forth. Therefore, this neurogenic inflammation occurs, causing the tissue to look red, feel itchy or painful, and cause a great deal of discomfort with penetration.

Neurogenic inflammation may also be the cause of increasingly severe pain and tissue reaction in and around the lesions of endometriosis. It is also now known among researchers that estrogen has an enhancing affect on this nerve-generated inflammation, which may partially explain why so many more women than men have chronic pain syndromes.

PROVIDING A BETTER UNDERSTANDING OF PAIN

These findings may also be the beginning of a better understanding of why pain syndromes experienced by women, such as migraine, fibromyalgia, and chronic pelvic pain, are made worse on a cyclic basis related to the menses.

In addition, Dr. Berkley's research with endometriosis has possibly given us an explanation as to why the signs and symptoms of this disorder often do not match up with the clinical findings. Doctors have long been puzzled as to why so many women with only tiny amounts of endometriosis can be in such pain and how other patients with very extensive endometriosis may experience no pain at all; the symptoms may depend on the new nerves in some lesions, rather than simply from the lesions themselves. Clearly there is an observational disconnect that now begins to make sense based on the results of Dr. Berkley's research and that has a far-reaching impact when applied to other pelvic pain issues.

SPEAKING THE LANGUAGE OF PAIN

Dr. Echenberg believes that patients must begin to understand the extensive cross-talk that is constantly occurring between not only the organs of the pelvis but between those organs and the surrounding muscles, ligaments, and skin in the pelvic region. If patients (and more doctors) get a grasp on these research findings, there will be a complete shift in how pelvic and sexual pain conditions are diagnosed and treated. Clinicians who see patients with any type of otherwise unexplained chronic pain in the pelvis should think about the possibility of these cross-connections of organs/tissues before making a definitive diagnosis about the pain or telling the patient that it's all in her head (and not in the way Dr. Berkley described!).

There are simple questions that a doctor can ask patients to best guide them to the correct diagnosis and treatment, but for this to happen, family doctors, gynecologists, and other specialists have to become willing to educate themselves. While it's impossible for any doctor to become expert in the entire body, Dr. Echenberg said:

> They need to learn at least a bit of neuroscience about the visceral organs (bladder, lower bowel, and reproductive) as well as the somatic tissues in the pelvis (muscles, nerves, ligaments, and skin) to recognize the signs of CPP. Aggressive treatment of the pain itself is vital, even if objective clinical findings at that moment are minimal or absent altogether, because my experience has proven time and again that pain generates more pain.

SEXUAL ABUSE AND PELVIC PAIN

Sexual abuse is one contributor to pelvic and sexual pain that must be acknowledged. A number of controlled studies have shown that women with CPP have a higher incidence of previous sexual and physical abuse than the general population.[4]

Dr. Gerig echoed Dr. Echenberg's notion of nervous system imprinting and related it to abuse: "I believe that there's memory in your cells. If you've been abused at some point in your life, when somebody pushes on that area, even if it's in a loving relationship, it makes sense that an abused woman would passively tense her pelvis and not want to let anyone in." Dr. Kahn agreed, giving as an example, "Think about women who deliver their babies vaginally. That's a terrible physical trauma, but usually associated with a wonderful psychological event. Compare that to a sexual assault, which is physical trauma associated with a terrible psychological event. It sets one up for the hypersensitivity that can lead to CPP."

AWARENESS, GUIDANCE, SUPPORT

Clinical psychologist and sex therapist Dr. Judy Kuriansky said that it's vital for women to be sensitive to all the sensations in their body: "Instead of panicking about pain, welcome it as a way to ask, 'What's going on with me?' I don't mean to welcome it in a happy way. But you can reduce any escalating anxiety by being sensitive to your body's sensations and what your body is telling you."

Julie Spencer, a pelvic floor physical therapist in Bethlehem, PA, believes that the most important task around chronic pelvic pain is making the public aware of the issue: "Women need to understand how common it is. We need to encourage them to seek treatment and reassure them that they are not alone. Their illness is not in their heads. There's help, guidance, and support available."

STILL A LONG WAY TO GO

While my research tells me there *is* growing support, it's slow going. Most sexual pain patients yearning for a diagnosis frequently see a host of doctors: family doctor, gynecologist, urologist, gastroenterologist, orthopedist, dermatologist, chiropractor, general pain management specialist, herbal and holistic practitioners, and, finally, the psychiatrist.

Most often, when doctors can't find an organic problem after multiple tests or surgery, they tend to dismiss the patient or send her to the next provider on the rung. Dr. Echenberg said, "Some doctors have confided in me that the patients they refer are ones they just don't want to see walking into their office one more time with phantom complaints. They've run out of ideas or they've surgically removed everything that might cause the pain. There's nothing else to take out."

Commonly, gynecologists are trained to think surgically, so if there isn't a lump or a bump, they don't believe their patients' complaints. However, Dr. John F. Steege, gynecologist, professor, and chief of the Advanced Laparoscopy and Pelvic Pain division, Department of Obstetrics and Gynecology at the University of North Carolina at Chapel Hill noted, "I do see encouraging changes. Many doctors are becoming attuned to the notion that just because it looks normal doesn't mean it feels normal to the patient."

Pain is a signal. Please don't ignore it. Seek help early and don't stop searching for answers until you get them. If you remember one thing from this chapter, it's this: Just because you can't see pain doesn't mean it isn't there.

LIVING WITH CPP: SUSAN'S JOURNAL

So, there you have it. We appear to be stuck with this albatross of a partner, CPP, an aggravating, annoying, agonizing palpable entity who refuses to move out. Like a vampire we've inadvertently invited in, CPP slowly sucks the life out of us, leaving a shell of a person behind, one who looks perfectly normal but is forever changed. Come to think of it, I've had toxic relationships with men that had similar results. Here is my own personal comparison.

With CPP, I started out just living my life, enjoying activities and skipping over bumps in the road that seemed short-lived. I didn't recognize the seriousness of the symptoms that were brewing. So, too, these relationships started out just fine, despite the little hints I didn't notice from the get-go.

With CPP, when I finally got socked with symptoms, I should have done something right then. Instead, I tried to tough it out, thinking things would get better soon. So, too, the first time the alcoholic boyfriend called me crying from some unknown location begging me to find him, I should have gotten out. The boyfriend who began criticizing my every word, becoming louder and increasingly nasty over time, should have had a short shelf life, but each time he pled for mercy, I weakened.

With CPP, over time I felt worse, but I adjusted my life accordingly to mitigate the pain, for instance, wearing looser pants or ensuring I always knew where there was a bathroom. As far as my relationships were concerned, I'd try not to make the angry boyfriend mad and stopped expecting the drunken boyfriend to show up for holidays or get the help he needed. I loved these guys in some very dysfunctional way and didn't want to let go. In both cases, I hoped and prayed for a miracle that would make the problems go away. Slowly, I became somewhat dead inside.

Finally, when the pain welled up to the point where I could no longer ignore it, I got fed up with both my CPP and these men. Regarding my pain syndrome, I began an unrelenting search for a diagnosis and help. With these losers, I finally got the courage to dump them and decided I would rather be alone than put up with all that mess.

After a number of years, I finally met my current husband, a gem of a man with flaws (uh, I have them too), who, as you will learn in this book is incredibly wonderful—and incredibly not! But overall, he's an A+ partner. I relish the great times, and we work through the bad ones. So it is, too, with my CPP.

Finally, I have to say that the best analogy I can make between CPP and men is to compare it to the relationship I have with my ex-husband, the father of my son. This relationship is also a chronic condition. I think the medical term is *pain in the ass,* which definitely corresponds to some of my CPP symptoms. Because we share a son, I will never totally escape our relationship. Like CPP, sometimes things are going quite well, but the "condition" endures, simmering beneath the surface. Eventually, the pain, rearing its ugly head, moves up the ladder to consciousness, with no way out until the agony subsides once again.

Chapter Five

SEXUAL PAIN AND OUR MOST INTIMATE RELATIONSHIPS

I wouldn't tell him when it hurt. "Suck it up princess," I told myself.

—Kat (interviewee)

Sometimes I let him finish because I felt badly for him, despite the fact that I rip, tear, bleed and sometimes have to take a week off work due to pain and the inability to walk, sit, and wear underwear or pants.

—Survey respondent

When the pain first started, I silently continued intercourse. When the pain was severe, I just had to stop. We would try at times, but I couldn't stand the pain. Eventually, my husband quit going to bed with me. He would stay up at night watching porn and satisfying his needs. He also talked on the phone late at night. I have plenty of clues he's had affairs, but I don't know for sure. We were married only two years when the pain started.

—Survey respondent

The physical therapist measured my husband's penis, and made a customized dilator to help me learn to accommodate him. Now, it's one thing to have something in your hand and use it, but a penis can only do so much. You can't take a penis off and say, "Okay, here we go." He's attached to it.

—Ellen (interviewee)

Sex. Pain-free, blissful sex. I want it. You want it. We miss it.

And that's what this chapter is about: what has happened to the sex lives of women who suffer with sexual pain and the partners who suffer along with them. Sex is an integral part of our lives, connected to the very life force itself, a basic instinct that's supposed to make us feel good. Instead, due to this deep-rooted illness, sex has become the bogeyman, a force to be feared instead of embraced.

Women too often suffer in silence, gritting their teeth, hiding their tears, and enduring the stabbing, burning, searing pain of intercourse, penetration, or other acts without breathing a word of this shameful syndrome to anyone. Or finally, pushed to the limit, a woman will just blurt out the truth to her partner, who is then forced to share the burden. In a world that worships sexual gratification, with volumes written on achieving the ultimate orgasm or turning up the heat in long-standing relationships, such a situation can tear a couple apart.

WHAT IS SEX?

I must admit, I've become especially confused about the definition of sex since writing this book. Not since hearing former President Bill Clinton say "I did not have sex with that woman" have I so deeply questioned what the term means. It seems that he wasn't the only one that didn't count oral sex or other intimate acts as the real thing.

The majority of interviewees for *Secret Suffering* used the word sex to mean intercourse. Of course intercourse is a form of sex. But to me, sex includes kissing, fondling, rubbing, touching, and oral stimulation. Surely masturbation is sex, so doing the same to someone else had to be sex too, right? And sharing an orgasm in whatever manner with someone you love seems intensely intimate to me.

Apparently, my interpretation isn't shared by all. Sex means whatever each partner, or the couple together, decides it means. Unfortunately, it was terribly sad to hear women or couples insist that, no matter how painful, sex had to include intercourse or it didn't count at all, so the end of the relationship was in sight because of shortsightedness.

SEXUAL PAIN: THE VISITOR THAT NEVER LEAVES

The pain sometimes begins slowly, an insidious deterioration of the fiber that binds couples. Sometimes, a sudden event inflames the fire so that both partners are stunned by the downward spiral of their intimacy to near nothingness.

Either way, eventually, the pain takes on a palpable presence, as if an ancient god to whom these mortals must bow and make sacrifice. Sometimes, the "Master" is beneficent, so the couple can freely express their love. At other times, like a tyrant with no mercy, each is pulled back, barely able to reach out and touch. The disorders that cause women to suffer pain in their private parts, the vagina, vulva, clitoris, labia, urethra, even the back and bowel, are an insidious lot, wreaking havoc on the intimacy that keeps couples close.

Gynecologist, and professor and chief of the Advanced Laparoscopy and Pelvic Pain division, Department of Obstetrics and Gynecology at the University of North Carolina at Chapel Hill Dr. John F. Steege's observation about sexual pain and relationships sums it up best:

> It goes without saying that pain issues impact relationships. Certainly if it goes on long enough, patients commonly get depressed, which becomes part of the illness as well.
>
> The metaphor I like to use with patients is that the pain becomes sort of a houseguest you thought was going to come for a little while and go away . . . and then never leaves.
>
> Somehow you have to incorporate that guest into your lives, into what used to be your relationship. But you always feel like you've got a third one there that you weren't counting on and that alters your conversation. If you can imagine it, there is always somebody listening to your conversations.
>
> Well, the illness is listening in a way. So you change what you say, and you avoid sensitive issues and you don't problem solve as well as you did before. You live a somewhat truncated emotional life that affects the individual and the couple profoundly.
>
> Couples recognize it at a certain level but they also say to themselves, "Well, gee, if only this pain would go away, we would be fine" when the reality is often otherwise. When the pain does go away, they find out they're not so fine because they haven't been paying attention to the relationship, in the usual ways, in front of this unwelcome guest.

Here's one of the problems: The woman suffers the pain, but the man suffers the consequences. He doesn't hurt, so it's often difficult for him to understand (or maybe even believe) that his partner *can't* have sex. He might think she's just making an excuse. And let's face it. How can your partner understand that his penis might feel like a human skewer? He can't possibly empathize with the torturous burning, stinging, or ripping feelings you experience.

As you'll hear from the women and men whose journeys we follow throughout *Secret Suffering*, nothing about sex and the pain is clear-cut. How to deal with sex in these relationships is a confusing issue involving a complex set of feelings.

SELF-SACRIFICE, ADJUSTMENT, OR NO SEX AT ALL

Most women tell of steeling themselves and allowing their partners to have intercourse with them at least some of the time, often turning their faces away so their partner can't see the pain. Every woman interviewed expressed guilt or an attitude of feeling sorry for her partner about denying him this particular pleasure.

However, one of the biggest surprises in writing *Secret Suffering* was discovering that most partners are tremendously supportive, yet the women who suffer often have painful sex anyway, when, in fact, their partners would not leave or cheat on them if they didn't. Of course, the skeptic in me whispers that maybe it's easy for men to be supportive when it's not inconvenient; it's easy to be supportive when the women succumbs to intercourse anyway despite the man's protestations that she doesn't have to do so.

I've interviewed couples who had no sexual contact at all for extended periods and the partner stayed by her side. There are couples who found ways to maintain the bonds between them on an emotional, spiritual, and physical level, despite the chronic pain. Some couples expressed the feeling that these issues have brought them closer.

In couples who have been together for 20 years or more, I found that both partners felt their history together overrode the difficult sexual component of their relationship. Long-time husband Gus, who was interviewed with his wife, Lois, had this to say: "I love her, and this condition is simply part of who she is. It's something I accept about her, and I try not to make it any more of a problem for her than it already is."

Most often, partners who succeeded in staying close were willing to experiment with other forms of sexual gratification and be satisfied with that level of intimacy, which goes back to the idea of thinking outside the box about what makes for gratifying sex.

While there *are* some women for whom any sexual contact is painful, even many of those have found ways to make their relationships sexually satisfying for their partners as they persisted in a determined effort to find relief. For the lucky ones, they respond to treatment and experience times where sex is pain-free and learn to ride the waves during a relapse.

The other surprise—an amusing one to me—was that no sex meant once a week for some and years for another. This was true of both women and men. So the amount of sex needed to sustain intimacy is apparently up for grabs. During my interviews with the unhappy once-a-weekers, I was reminded of the Woody Allen movie *Annie Hall*. In a scene that had the audience roaring with universal recognition, they were at their respective therapists' offices, recounting the details of their strained sex life. To paraphrase:

Her: "It's just awful. He wants sex all the time. It's like once a week."
Him: "It's a nightmare. We barely have sex at all. Just once a week."

LOIS'S DOWNWARD SPIRAL INTO PAIN

Lois is in her early 60s. She's been married to Gus for over 40 years. Lois has vulvodynia and pudendal nerve neuropathy. She remembers the exact moment her problems began. "I was walking on a boardwalk in Ocean City, New

Jersey, in 1994 and stumbled a little. A pain hit me and I just thought my underwear was too tight. I waited a couple of weeks to see the doctor. He said I had tendonitis, gave me some pain pills, and sent me on my way."

She continued to suffer with "a burning, blow-torch type of pain." The pain was aggravated by wearing fitted clothing, walking, climbing stairs, bending, and even sitting. Lying down was the only way to relieve the pain.

Before the boardwalk incident, Lois and her husband had sex once every two weeks, and were satisfied with that. But she said that once the pain began, "the gate closed."

Over the weeks, the pain increased to the point where they simply couldn't have intercourse at all. She said, "It came on just that fast! I think at that point it wasn't so much the vulvodynia as it was the vaginal nerves. When I started going to doctors, I couldn't stand to have them even touch me down there." And 23 years later, her vaginal nerves were still so raw that Dr Echenberg couldn't put the tip of a Q-tip on her genital area the first time he saw her.

Lois's husband, Gus, also vividly remembers that day on the boardwalk, the day their lives were inexorably changed. He said, "It was so sudden. Yeah, we thought it was just a pulled muscle. And then it just never went away." The pain began to interfere with their sex life shortly after the incident. Gus said, "It really took me back. I remember thinking, 'What am I doing wrong?' and she assured me, 'No, no, no. It's not you! I don't know what it is.'"

Lois was lucky. She had a supportive husband who would stand by her over the years. But there are other, less understanding men who get angry because they believe that their partner is simply withholding sex. Mirriam was married to one such man.

MIRRIAM'S FRUSTRATION

Mirriam, a young mother from Costa Rica, said her pain was minimal when she first married, but as the discomfort increased, her relationship disintegrated. At first, during intercourse, her vagina felt "extra dry." She said, "In the beginning, you know, you have sex all the time! But during the second or third time, I was so dry, it was painful."

As the years went on and the pain increased, her desire for sex diminished greatly, but she still wanted to please her husband. Once, when they were drunk, they had anal sex, but because she also had hemorrhoids, the pain was unbearable.

Mirriam also had bladder pressure, but the pressure turned to severe pain in her back in addition to the vaginal burning and bowel pressure during sex. She said, "It was so painful I would just tell my husband to 'take it out.' Thankfully, he would finish really fast. I was happy about that."

Mirriam told me her husband would sometimes withhold money when she wanted something. "He'd say, 'Do you think you really deserve it?' But what he was trying to tell me was, 'You haven't had sex with me in a long time, so you don't really deserve anything.' I felt like he was saying, 'You aren't good to me, so I'm not going to be good to you.'" Eventually, she left her husband.

Mirriam's case is extreme, but Dr. Lyndsay Elliott, clinical psychologist, believes a lot of frustration builds between couples when the woman suffers with CPP "in terms of not feeling good enough, not feeling capable enough, not being able to communicate well." She said partners have difficulty understanding where the other is coming from. "There's a lot of fear in terms of sexual engagement and then frustration from the partner's point of view if they can't engage."

NOT MUCH APPRECIATION FROM MALE PARTNERS

"Most males don't have an appreciation for the debility the women are experiencing. And they are usually uneducated about why this is happening." That opinion was expressed by the late Dr. C. Paul Perry, gynecologist and medical director for the C. Paul Perry Pelvic Pain Center in Birmingham, Alabama, who added, "There are definitely marriages broken up by this issue. Most patients have made every effort to rectify the problem but just haven't been able to get the right medical attention. But we encourage the family to come in with the patient because most times the patient is misunderstood, especially by the husband."

Lois said that without her husband's supportive attitude, "We would not have survived. He would have been gone if he hadn't been understanding. I think some men just don't want to understand the complexity of the problem, and that's why divorces and separations can happen as a result."

Patients commonly bring their partners with them to doctors' appointments. But why do they come in? Is it voluntary? Is it because they want to find out if their partners are really suffering as they describe? Or do they truly want to be part of the solution? According to Dr. Steege, there may be a variety of reasons:

> When you go into the room and the partner is sitting there reading a magazine while you're talking to the patient, it may appear they're uncomfortable being in that environment. We do see that at times. Part of that behavior is anxiety. Part of it is being in strange territory. They may not know what to do with themselves. Partners feel all sorts of emotions about the situation, just as patients do. It's important to include the partner in the conversation because it's not just the patient who is suffering. We have to value his feelings and let him be heard.

Dr. Echenberg agreed and added that he has seen a variety of reactions from partners when they come in for visits. Many are supportive, but he's seen a number of partners who seemed embarrassed about exposing their intimacy to strangers. He added that there are some partners who come in and take over the conversation, answering all the questions, and exhibiting overt controlling behaviors. Sometimes, the partner won't go to the doctor at all, which compounds the communications problem and may increase doubts about whether the patient is really being honest.

Lois's husband is a perfect example of this problem. For a long time, he wouldn't go with Lois to the doctor, so off she'd go, only to be disappointed time and time again.

Still, Gus pushed her to continue her search. When she'd come home in tears with stories about what doctors said and how they treated her, he was astonished, sometimes saying, "Well, that's not possible." Eventually, he became skeptical about her perception of the experience.

Finally, Lois insisted he learn first-hand, and Gus went with Lois to a renowned women's center in a neighboring state. That was the beginning of their partnership in the battle against sexual pain. She told me about Gus's epiphany. "After we left the office, he said, 'I know what you're saying now. They didn't even examine you.' They undressed me, sat me on a table, asked me questions, then told me I could get dressed."

Her husband was livid at the treatment his wife received and confronted one of the doctors, saying, "Don't you need to examine her?" The doctor replied, "No, we can deal with it based on what she's told us."

Gus told me he felt defeated. "I finally understood what she'd been trying to tell me. It was absolutely ridiculous for us to travel all that distance for them to basically say, 'Okay, here's some reading material.' It was an insult." Since then, Lois's husband has been her staunchest advocate.

Eventually, Lois and Gus found Dr. Echenberg and the help she needed. Gus went with Lois to physical therapy and learned how to massage her internal vaginal muscles. Lois explained that going through the process together drew them closer. "He saw me lying on a gynecologist's table and could tell as soon as the doctor touched me how painful it was. He got involved in understanding how comprehensive this pain was. He's done a lot to help me try to solve this problem."

VALERIE HELPED BY PHYSICAL THERAPY

Valerie has PBS/IC, vestibulitis, and problems with her psoas muscle. Like Lois and Gus, she and her husband partnered to help her heal and worked together with a physical therapist (PT). Before having sex, Valerie's husband uses the internal massage technique they learned from the PT. Valerie explained:

> Of course, the PT would have a glove on and feel if the muscles inside were tense or relaxed. She'd massage the tense ones a little. So he'll do that. He can tell which ones are tense now. He'll use a little K-Y jelly and pulsate those muscles to loosen them up. If we do that first, it's so much better because I'm more relaxed and it doesn't hurt the whole time he's inside of me.

Not every man will participate to this extent. As one interviewee said of her unwilling husband, "He doesn't want to think of it as clinical." For the most part, I do think it's easier for men to be supportive when it's not inconvenient for them, or when they can remain passive observers because they know we'll give in just often enough that they aren't impacted by our pain too much. But if both partners do their part to help in the healing, they are sharing the burden and, most importantly, ensuring *she* enjoys sex too, so he's not having the pleasure at her expense.

MEN ARE PROBLEM SOLVERS

I've often heard that men want to solve problems, and if they can't fix it, they become frustrated. Sitting by and feeling helpless while they see their partners suffer with pelvic pain is quite difficult for many men.

Gus is just such a man. Lois said, "My husband deals with numbers in his job, but with pelvic pain, it's just not cut and dried. He believes there's a solution to every problem because of his mathematical background. It's difficult for him to comprehend why something can't be done about my sexual pain."

Lois stressed that if you are married or in a relationship and suffer from this condition, urge your husband or partner to seek help with you until you both find answers. Men may not want to get involved with the intricacies of these issues, but, as Lois said, "Until they deal with it, they'll never understand how you're affected by the pain."

This struck me as a key point, because whether they like it or not, it's to the man's benefit to do everything possible to help his partner find relief, or he will suffer a nightmare of deprivation and the destruction of intimacy with his partner. However, even when partners are present and invested in trying to help, it's still often difficult for them to fully grasp the magnitude of the problem. Urologist Dr. Nel Gerig gave this example:

> I have a young patient with pelvic pain who comes in with her boyfriend. She says, "I'm not normal. I don't know that I'll ever be able to have a normal life. This is so unfair."
>
> Her boyfriend is clearly supportive because he comes with her to every appointment. But every time, he asks, "When can we have sex? When's it not going to hurt?" He'll say, "If she just tried to have it more, that would help her, right? If she were just willing to try . . ."

Dr. Gerig pulls no punches to bring him back to reality and suggest how he can help her *and* their relationship, "No. That won't help her. Get over it. Go take a cold shower." Dr. Gerig added, "My goal for her is to have sex like a wild woman and have it not hurt as soon as possible. But not today! So you'll have to wait, and in the meantime explore other avenues to achieve intimacy."

Gus, Lois's husband, explains the attitude of young men such as the one Dr. Gerig described, saying, "It doesn't affect me as much as it does her because she lives with it 24 hours a day, whereas I only see it when she's in obvious pain or when we want to have sex." However, even though Lois says her husband is as supportive a man as you'll find, she admitted, "He still tries to have intercourse. He still acts like I can." And she laughed.

Her off-handed comment seemed a profound statement about men who love women with pelvic pain, men like my husband, who tries his best to be understanding and compassionate. But in our intimate moments, my husband, too, tries again and again to have intercourse, even when I've made it clear that it's a burn time. I get annoyed, surprised, and sometimes just want to scream, "How can you possibly ask for that?" And then, sometimes I just give in because I feel bad for him, or because it's easier than arguing about it.

But maybe it's not that men are thick-headed, boorish beasts, thinking only of themselves. After all, as Gus said, *they* are not in pain. Is it possible that they truly love us, are not deliberately inconsiderate, but in that moment want fervently to believe that we are well, that we *can* have sex? Or maybe it's just a genetic instinct that drives them to forget.

Lois agreed and jokingly explained her personal theory: "I do think it's in their male genes. They're just predisposed to be that way. I think it's the old male idea of 'Let's go to bed. Let's do it. Boom, boom, boom.' Even though they know you're in pain, they still forget and think, 'Oh maybe we can just do it. Let's just go do it right now.' But for me, I can't. I can't do it."

LAUREN CAN'T JUST SAY NO

Lauren's story bears out my theory about men who are supportive when the price isn't too high, the denial of women about the severity of their pain, and having the courage to "just say no." However, she also exemplifies a woman trying to find ways to be intimate without drowning in pain.

Lauren suffers with vulvar vestibulitis. She's been married almost 37 years and said she has a wonderful marriage. Her pain began two years before our interview. She told me she simply "puts up" with painful intercourse without telling her husband it hurts when they are in bed. She feels he *deserves* intercourse and doesn't want him to feel guilty, but she clearly suffers, saying:

> It hurts so much afterward, I wouldn't be anxious to do it again the next day. But typically I wouldn't tell him. I don't know if that's being dishonest. I mean, it's perseverance. On the other hand, if there's something I can do to shorten the process, I will.
>
> I know he loves me. I know he would never do anything to hurt me. Life has not been all happiness and wonder. There have been some difficult times and we

somehow managed to get through them and, in all reality, this is not the worst thing that's ever happened to me.

Lauren insisted that she and her husband work through their sexual issues outside of the bedroom, so this disease hasn't negatively impacted their overall relationship. She told me:

> My husband is appropriately demanding, and we do our talking outside of the actual act of sex. He knows I burn every day, and he's supportive of all the therapies I've done. We've just learned to accommodate, and sex might be a little less frequent, but it's not zero. It's never ever been zero.
>
> I'm not averse to trying different things. Sometimes I apply ice ahead of time, even a glass of water with ice cubes in it between my legs. I can just sit with it for 15 or 20 minutes, and that seems to calm the burning down. We read each other so well that we don't put the other in a difficult situation very often. I also let him know when I have a zero burn day, so he's very much aware of the fact that "Okay, today's the day for sex."

Lauren finds that the missionary position puts too much pressure on her, so she prefers to be on top. She said, "I really can't handle the force of him on top banging into my pubic bone."

Outside the bedroom, Lauren is one of many women who find standing up more comfortable than sitting. When she's standing or walking, she doesn't feel the burn. But when she sits, a tightness, often from restricted clothing, seems to aggravate her condition, like cutting off her circulation. "And if I don't know what to do to relieve the pressure," she said, "I take a bath for half an hour. That usually calms it down a little bit."

She finds water neutral and sensual, saying, "I can orgasm with the shower massage and have sex right after that. It makes the process go a whole lot faster." Often, her husband participates with her in the shower, but she explained, "I also have a vibrator I can use in the water so I can control the touch. It's a lot better than just squirming and wincing at his touch, which is not necessarily gentle. I might pull his hand away because he's out of control." Every woman has her threshold, and while it's sad that sex should serve up any pain at all, knowing where the grey areas begin and end make a big difference.

Thankfully, great moments still happen for women who have learned how to manage their sexual pain, moments when their sexual experience is exquisite once again. Lauren recounted one such time:

> We went out to dinner and both smelled like smoke because we were in a restaurant that allowed smoking. I rinsed my hair out and slipped into bed without anything on. When my husband got into bed, he was totally surprised and excited by my nudity. I said, "I'll do anything you want." We had a really great time. He penetrated me and it was fine, and we fell asleep happily ever after.

Lauren would be happy to satisfy her husband with oral sex even on a burn day. But when she offers, her husband would rather wait until they can both "do something," referring to intercourse. She said, "If I just can't, I'll tell him, 'You know I love you and want to make you feel good.' But then we end up doing nothing, which makes me feel guilty and both of us feel frustrated, or I give in and feel resentful, but he's happy. This disease sucks."

MEN'S SELF-ESTEEM IS DIMINISHED

A man's feelings of self-worth are also diminished by this unwelcome guest. Dr. Gerig pointed out the effect a woman's sexual pain has on the man's self-esteem. "Sometimes they can't have intercourse for long periods of time," she said, "so the husband will say to the wife 'you don't love me anymore.' He takes it as a rejection. A lot of married couples have difficulty discussing their intimacy and sexual activity in the first place. Add the interplay between the psychological aspects, the pain aspects, and the medical aspects of what is happening to the woman, and you've exponentially compounded the difficulties."

Lois's husband, Gus, has accepted the situation, albeit grudgingly, saying:

> Obviously I want intercourse a lot more. But these are the cards we've been dealt. We get around it and she's very good about it. Sometimes she pleases me without my doing anything for her.
> Sometimes I can't bring her to orgasm but she makes me come and says she's satisfied. It's obviously not a complete act, but that's what happens most of the time. The times we have intercourse are very few and far between. But I do consider it sex, even if it's not intercourse.

So Lois's husband is accepting of other sexual avenues with his wife, but clearly, he doesn't seem happy about it. He said, "It's true that it gets a little frustrating, but over the course of all these years, I'm getting immune to it and just take advantage of the times we can have sex."

A GUESSING GAME

I have to say that it's somewhat unfair to be angry at our partners if we don't tell them that we're in pain when having intercourse or other sexual activity. After all, we may be close in many ways, but really, can they read our minds? Gus loves Lois, but that doesn't make him a mind reader. I guess my husband isn't either.

Gus can't tell if Lois is hurting during intercourse unless he feels her wince and pull away or she point blank tells him. "If that happens," he said, "I can try not going so deep, but most times we have to stop intercourse. Of course, I don't love that, but every time it happens, she has, you know, got me off. She says, 'I'm not going to take it out on you' and I tell her that it's not necessary, but it's what almost always happens."

Lois will sometimes let Gus manually stimulate her, even when his touch hurts her because she feels his frustration about their inability to have intercourse. "It helps him feel manly," she said. "I think many women put up with a lot so their husbands get some satisfaction out of the act." But Gus *wants* to give back. When she can't reach orgasm, he feels awful. "I tell him it's not his fault," said Lois. "But he takes it personally when he can't satisfy me. I tell him to just rub my back and I'll be fine. I get as much satisfaction out of a back rub as sex. So he's kind of gotten used to it."

LIVING WITH CPP: SUSAN'S JOURNAL

I laughed when Lois mentioned back rubs because they're pure pleasure for me, too. No fear of pain, a constant stream of heightened sensation. Now that I've heard another woman say she feels exactly the same way, I wonder if this is an epidemic, too.

I once came up with a great plan for Jay and I to schedule time on Sundays for intimacy. It worked well for us—for the few months we stayed committed to it. I knew if we didn't schedule it, I'd come up with excuse after excuse based on my fear of pain. I knew it was a good thing in any event because, with our busy lives, we could go weeks without spending *any* kind of quality time together, much less having sex.

Like it or not, want it or not, into the bed we'd go. We'd snuggle for awhile, talk, and giggle, and inevitably we'd end up having some type of sexual activity, I'd even have an orgasm most of the time, and I'd always get my anxiously awaited back rub. A middle-aged friend of mine, one who doesn't experience sexual pain, put it best, "Sex is like cleaning the toilet. You hate doing it, but boy, do you feel better afterward." Yep, I think that about summed it up for me.

I'd like to say there's a happy ending to this story, but somehow, our Sunday schedule fell away. Life got busy. Sex hurt more. My libido diminished further. We were both stressed out and tired. It does seem easier to ignore it all, but what happens is that the dirt piles up and we tend to argue more often about ridiculous things. Truth be told, I don't clean my toilet much either.

SO, *IS* INTERCOURSE THE ONLY SEX THAT COUNTS?

The big question stays with me: Is intercourse the only sex that counts? We don't want to be alone, and we don't want the guilt of not pleasing our partners. It was apparent that most of the people with whom I spoke felt that any other sexual activity was the poor stepsister who didn't get to go to the ball. Despite the fact that, according to Dr. Gerig, there is a small population of women who hurt when touched anywhere, for the majority, oral sex, mutual masturbation, vibrators, and so forth, work great. Even if women have sensitivity in those areas, they know how to get around that. So why does it make any difference how you have sex, especially if it doesn't hurt? Why wouldn't you and your partner still feel close and satisfied? It seems that for those of us who can't have traditional sex without pain, thinking outside the box is vital to healing our intimate relationships.

To me, it's like giving birth. When I was pregnant, I wanted to have a completely natural delivery, with midwives, music, Lamaze, the works. But when my son was breech and just wouldn't budge, I had to have a C-section. I felt a twinge of disappointment and inferiority because of the emphasis on natural being the best way (further reinforced by the smug, judgmental, condescending attitude of some mothers who had given birth through their vaginal canal). Sam's now turning 18. The bottom line was that I had a healthy baby boy (though now an obnoxious, feral teenager), so did it really matter how he was born? As far as I'm concerned, it should be the same with sex.

I asked Dr. Gerig why most men (and some women) don't consider other types of sex equally fulfilling. She responded, "Patients with erectile dysfunction face the same issue. I tell these men the real issue is intimacy, not physical, sexual intercourse."

Dr. Judy Kuriansky, clinical psychologist and sex therapist, weighed in on this issue:

> Intercourse is such a traditionally ingrained idea. It's very hard to change people's thinking. There are reasons why women might resist putting other sexual behaviors in the same realm of importance because they think of them as less intimate.
>
> For example, some women may think that oral sex means they're not equal or being treated as respectfully or that they're as intimate with their partners as they would be with intercourse.
>
> Deeper emotional attachments and meanings are associated with the act of intercourse, and that's why it persists as being significant. And anthropologically, people have that ingrained idea genetically.

What Valerie Does When it Hurts

Valerie has been married five years and with her husband for almost eight. They are now in their early 30s. She has interstitial cystitis, vulvar vestibulitis, and spasms in her psoas muscle. Her pain began shortly after they got married.

> We talk about everything, so he knew I was having problems because, obviously, when I'm having problems, we can't have sex as often. We don't have sex very often

right now, maybe once every two weeks, but we do other things sexually. He's pretty laid back about the whole thing.

Valerie said that her husband is fine if she tells him to stop in the middle of intercourse because he doesn't want to hurt her. Then she said something I found odd, but in line with the attitude of so many women I spoke to who suffered with CPP, including me. "When we're having intercourse, I'll tell him if it's bothering me, but usually I want to work through the pain. Sometimes it hurts at first but not later. So he'll say, 'Do you want to stop?' and I'll tell him, 'Well let me see if I feel better.'"

Though I didn't comment, I felt the sadness of knowing that Valerie felt compelled to "work through the pain." And of course, before she tells him to stop (if and when she does), he's going at it, *not* feeling deprived. Like Gus, Valerie's husband is not uncaring but probably oblivious to her pain because she hides it so well. As a woman who has *not* spoken up more times than I care to count during sex/intercourse, I know the confused emotions and guilt that can surround sex and pain and feeling responsible for someone else's pleasure. I also know from experience that sometimes intercourse doesn't hurt as much as at other times and that sometimes the pain *does* lessen with each thrust. How tragic it is that this most intimate act, one that is supposed to be pure pleasure, has become so mixed with suffering and endurance for women like us. Sheer pleasure? Hardly.

Not Having Sex Doesn't Cut it with Jane

Jane is a 40-year-old woman who was diagnosed with painful bladder syndrome, otherwise known as interstitial cystitis (PBS/IC). Her experience with sexual pain began in 1993 with "shooting pains" in her vagina. The pain was intermittent, so it didn't really disrupt Jane and her husband's sex life—not at first. Gradually, the pain became more insistent until she couldn't have sex at all during flare-ups. Her husband is very supportive, but he won't let her satisfy him when she isn't up to full-blown sex. She's devastated by his attitude.

Sometimes she can't tolerate orgasms because they set off internal muscle spasms and make her feel worse. She finds it very disturbing that her husband will not allow her to sexually please him during those times. She told him that it would give her the measure of intimacy she desperately craved and said, "I feel that if I'm pleasing him and we're holding each other, we're intimate and it's fine with me. But he doesn't buy it. He said, 'If it's not mutual, it's not much of an experience.'"

But for Jane, *not* having sex in some form with her husband is simply not an option. "It's ripping away any shred of self-esteem I might still have. It makes me feel like shit that he's just not interested."

Jane recently bought some sex toys to help stimulate their sex life. "He hasn't seen the toys yet. I bought something called a masturbating sleeve, which is supposed to make it easier for me to use my hands. I was embarrassed as hell to be buying them. I ordered them on the Internet and I was still embarrassed."

Clearly, Jane urgently wants to strengthen her bond with her husband and convince him to open up to other ways she can express her love with him. She still has trepidation about her husband's possible reaction to the toys, saying, "I just wish I was sure he felt happy that I want to be close to him. I feel confident our marriage is going to last, but we are much less happy than we were."

In Jane's case, her love for her husband and desire to revive their intimacy overcame her embarrassment. We have to be champions of the cause, even when our partners may have given up. There are so many paths to intimacy, we just need to be creative and open to them and help our partners reach that point as well.

Unfortunately, there are some men who don't care whether you enjoy sex. But the men who do care—who don't want to feel selfish—need to understand that we want to please them even when we can't have the pleasure reciprocated. When we suffer with sexual pain, our femininity is decimated. We may not be able to function sexually ourselves, but we still crave the emotional intimacy and connection.

Pauline Stood Her Ground and Said No

Pauline has vulvar vestibulitis and an ex-husband who didn't care about his wife's pain. She's in her mid-30s now, but her symptoms began when she was 15. She told me, "My husband would say, 'We never have sex,' and I'd tell him, 'We don't have sex because it hurts. But it's not like we don't have sexual relations.' Because oral and other forms of sex were not a problem for me."

Her ex-husband was well aware of her condition, but he did nothing to ease her mind. Before she finally got fed up and left him, she'd let her guilt override the pain during intercourse and wouldn't ask him to stop:

> I would say, "Alright, fine. I'm just gonna relax and you can do your thing and be done." He never really showed me one way or another if he cared or if he was just happy to be getting some. It was frustrating! So many times I'd cry afterwards because I'd be embarrassed about it, and he'd just say, "I'm going to sleep now."

Pauline's ex-husband made her life miserable when she wouldn't give in to his constant insistence on having intercourse. Unlike some women, however, she learned to stand her ground. She told me, "We'd be in bed and he'd say, 'Please, come on, why can't I have it?' and I'd say, 'Because it freakin' hurts. Get away from me.' Ultimately, I figured if he's begging me for it knowing it hurts me, then he probably doesn't care if I'm in pain." Intercourse became a contentious issue, and after an incessant battle, she finally just cut him off. "I told him he wasn't allowed to do that anymore, and after about three years of marriage, we got divorced. That issue was definitely one of the contributing factors, but it wasn't the only problem. We fought a lot, too."

There's a tremendous tug-of-war between pain and guilt for women with sexual pain who dread the thought of having sex and the anxiety or conflict that will inevitably ensue. Dr. Kuriansky agreed, stating two components of the problem: "One is the woman's own feelings and the other is how she expects her partner will respond. In some cases, as you describe, husbands and boyfriends will roll over the partner's resistance. Ultimately, she's afraid he'll leave her or have an affair if she doesn't do what he wants."

Dr. Perry added his thoughts, "In an attempt to preserve their relationships, women will sometimes try to mask their discomfort, especially during intercourse. Unfortunately, that just leads to more and more of a dysfunctional relationship and a lack of openness and honesty in their marriage."

LIVING WITH CPP: SUSAN'S JOURNAL

I just took a break from writing and went downstairs. It's been weeks since Jay and I had any type of sexual intimacy. We talked for a few minutes about the book, which led to more pointed references to sex. I told him I know he needs it. To my surprise, I actually wanted to have sex, too. But I also said I didn't want to feel pressured to have intercourse. I think my exact words were, "It's burning like the devil, so don't even think about putting it in."

For me, the real pain begins with intercourse. I'm sensitive in other areas, but "stick a fork in me, and I'm done." Jay doesn't want to hurt me, and he makes sure I have an orgasm first. But every single time, after I'm finished and when he's beginning to get fired up, he'll whisper to me that we should try, that he really wants it. But I don't want to try, because I can't remember the last time it didn't hurt at all, when I felt pure pleasure. And almost always, afterwards, I wear a medal of pain.

When he starts to whine and beg, I'm faced with pain or guilt. Sometimes I feel bad for him and mumble, "Okay"—an obvious, transparent lie—hoping and praying it won't hurt too much and will end soon, or even that maybe, just maybe, it won't hurt this time.

To Jay's credit, as he enters, he does ask if it hurts. If I can bear it, I'll say it doesn't hurt. And, in truth, sometimes, I actually can relax into it, though I *always* start out tensing up in anticipation of pain. Most of the time now, that tension is warranted, because it hurts badly, really, really badly. After he's satisfied and while he's still inside of me—as I'm blanketed with the afterglow of agony, wanting to scream "get the hell out of me!"—he asks once more if it hurt. At that point, I'll finally blurt out the truth as I shove him off of me. He always responds, "You should have told me. I would have stopped." And

I think to myself, "You shouldn't have asked to do it at all." But I know that's really unfair; ultimately it's *my* responsibility to say no to pain.

Even if it wasn't too painful during the act, afterward my vagina invariably throbs as if it's a time bomb ready to explode. Sometimes it feels like sharp shrapnel from an explosion going deep into me. After sex, it's peeing, peeing, peeing until, drop by drop, I finally finish—for the moment. Then I often go on a peeing spree, every 10 or 15 minutes for an hour. Sometimes going for "real," sometimes going by drops.

Even on those blissful occasions when intercourse doesn't burn as if his penis is on fire, or feel as if a knife is stabbing and punishing me, the myalgia, or muscular pain, lasts the rest of the day. (I love the sound of the word myyaaalllll-ggggiiiiiaaa because it sounds like what it feels like: a long, agonizing groan.)

I walk bow-legged out of the bathroom afterward, agony written across my face, moaning as quietly as possible, but by then he's usually on to something else. After all, it's my pain. I once asked him after having sex how he'd feel if his penis burned like a hot poker every time he had intercourse. He just said he couldn't imagine it and then gave me that back rub I love, which always feels good.

THE STICKY ISSUE OF FIDELITY

Gus, Lois's husband, was adamant about the importance of fidelity. In fact, he wanted to convey this strong message for men in relationships with women who suffer from CPP:

> An affair is not an option. Her sexual pain isn't a good reason. Obviously, I've thought about an affair. We've even talked about it. She might say something like, "Oh boy, you should just go out and get some!" No, no, you absolutely can't do that!

Jane's View on Fidelity

Jane confessed she and her husband no longer sleep in the same bed because she often wakes up nine times or more to pee, and her husband is a light sleeper. She believes that if the physical intimacy isn't there and you're not even sleeping in the same bedroom, the *emotional* intimacy drains out of your marriage. "I don't know why my husband hasn't left me, but when I asked him, he said, 'Are you going to leave *me?*' I said, 'No,' and he replied, 'Well, I'm not going to leave you either, so let's just take that off the table.'"

Ellen's View on Fidelity

Ellen told her husband that he should have an affair, but that she didn't want to know about it. She said his response was forceful:

He said, "You're crazy! I don't want that. If I wanted that I would have been gone!"

I say it's not fair to him. But men have ways of satisfying themselves by masturbating. That's part of their life. It doesn't matter if they're with someone. They do it anyway, whether they admit it or not. They can't help it. So they get that relief. But that's only one way of getting relief, because men also need intimacy. And sex *is* intimacy for men.

THE ULTIMATE MEASURE OF INTIMACY

Dr. Daniel Brookoff, oncologist and director of the Center for Medical Pain Management at Presbyterian-St. Luke's Medical Center in Denver, Colorado, told me patients come to him feeling invalidated. Some even say they'd rather have cancer because at least people would believe something was wrong. He stressed that someone may temporarily feel better being listened to and validated, but that won't help with the relationship, as this story indicated:

> I had a new patient today who took three hours to tell me her story. I just sat there and listened. I took notes. At the end, the patient said, "Thank you so much." I replied, "I didn't do anything." And the patient said, "No, you listened to me. You understand me."
>
> "No, I don't understand you," I said. "And I'm going to tell you something. I'm here to help you get better, not to understand you. We're going to do everything we can to get you better. But when you get better, you'll still find nobody's going to understand your condition."
>
> Patients have to realize that's not the point. Compare it to drowning. As you're drowning, you don't cry, "Nobody understands me!" You don't want to be understood. That's not going to help you. What you want is to be better.
>
> This idea of being understood disrupts relationships. Because what are you really trying to get out of a relationship? You're trying to help each other grow and make each other feel safe and welcome in this world. We have to help people focus on that and give them techniques to do that; otherwise they grow apart.

Dr. Brookoff encourages patients to bring their partners on their visits. When both partners are sitting in front of him, he says to the patient, "Your husband's job is not to understand you because he's not going to. His job is to love you and believe you, and if he and the rest of your family loves you and believes you, they're doing the best they can."

LIVING WITH CPP: SUSAN'S JOURNAL

The couples with whom I've spoken who have 30, 40, even 50 years of marriage talk about bonds that are stronger than sex. One husband said, "Our history together includes other things that make our life together worth it." I asked if he ever thought about having an affair. He said, "Well, I think about it, and she tells me I should, but I love her."

My own husband firmly responded to my suggestion of finding a mistress by saying, "You can't make my decision for me. Don't tell me what I want." The fact is, it's not so easy to find a good partner with whom to walk this difficult journey through life. Everyone has challenges to face, but often our sexuality is at the core of our self-image as women, so this situation is a problem of epic proportions.

My suggestion to my husband about getting a mistress may tumble out with burning tears and pain immediately following a sexual encounter that left me feeling particularly devastated and hopeless, or calmly, but resolutely, in the kitchen at some unsuspecting moment. I wonder if I suggest Jay find someone else so I don't have to deal with sex anymore, or if it's because I feel badly for him.

Pushing your significant other away while you work through issues doesn't mean you have to get rid of him forever. Jay's theory is that it's more important to be committed to the relationship than to each other because there are going to be hard times, tough breaks, and annoying moments. Even the best marriages suffer from disputes and pressure—financial, emotional, parenting, and so forth. Plenty of couples deal with other conditions such as paralysis, where sexuality may be severely affected, and still maintain strong bonds of love.

Remembering your bigger commitment will keep you from destroying the whole because of a problem in the moment or a mood or an argument. Sexual pain may ebb and flow, so there may be times of great intimacy and, yes, times when you can't even stand the sound of your partner breathing, much less his coming near you. But embracing Jay's philosophy can help you ride the waves until you reach the shore, instead of drowning in the sea.

Chapter Six

BILL: SEXUAL PAIN FROM A HUSBAND'S POINT OF VIEW

Bill is very much in love with his wife, Jackie, who looks like she's in her late 30s rather than her late 50s. They've been together over 25 years. Together, they have three adult children. However, the stress of the intimacy issues that have increased over the life of their marriage have made him question whether to stay or leave. To this day, Jackie has never been given a diagnosis for the continuing sexual pain she's suffered for most of those 25 years, nor does she seek medical treatment any longer for the physical pain.

For several years, Bill and his wife have been unable to have intercourse. Jackie is too afraid to even try due to the memory of the pain. He said, "Recently, with a heavy dose of wine, I did manage to get about halfway inside her for the first time in at least five years. But she couldn't take it. The irritation, the burning, was just so bad that she had to push me out."

FROM VIRGINITY TO PAIN

Bill was 32 when he met Jackie, who was 23, a virgin, and living at home. He had been married previously and dated quite a lot. Bill said they consummated their relationship after dating for six months. In the beginning, no problems were apparent; in fact, according to Bill they had a satisfying sex life. But problems crept in once they were married, even on their honeymoon, as Bill described:

> It seemed Jackie couldn't deal with frequency of sex. If we made love two days in a row, as newlyweds might, that would irritate her. She felt burning. So I'd say, "OK,

why don't we put a day in between?" And soon thereafter, two days, and then three. We kept working at how much recuperation time she needed before that tissue was less sensitive.

Eventually, she stopped wanting to put on a nice nightgown or negligee, fearful of even starting the activity. Even if I initiated sex, there was a good chance I would be rejected.

Once after her husband ejaculated inside of her, Jackie's vagina burned so badly, she sat in a bathtub trying to wash it out. Due to incidents such as this, over the next four years, Jackie developed even more apprehension at the thought of having sex. If Bill were romantic or playful, she would divert his attention and put up barriers by changing the mood. "We might fight over something we normally wouldn't, so there'd be no fooling around because we were mad at each other. I eventually realized Jackie was instigating these fights."

Bill told me that he could actually feel the texture inside of her vagina change to sandpaper during intercourse and described it like this:

> I would know to pull out by the change inside. I mean, I always pulled out if I felt it. She did begin feeling safer in knowing that I didn't want to hurt her, so she could tell me even before I knew it. After a while, she was willing to say, "I'm not doing well. Please pull out." I could tell every time we had intercourse in the early years whether it was going to go OK or not within the first three or four minutes.

Bill told me his wife saw at least 15 gynecologists—some of the best in the field, from heads of hospitals to departments of gynecology and obstetrics. They'd take biopsies of the skin and found nothing. Or they'd tell her she had a yeast infection. Sometimes they were right. More often, they were wrong. Every time she suffered another disappointing medical experience, Bill would continue to research and convince her to try again. Jackie resisted, saying, "But we've already been to 10 doctors." The numbers and costs continued to add up.

GOING FROM BAD TO WORSE

Then a new symptom developed. Her vaginal wall toward the perineum began to tear at the slightest attempt to enter, even no more than the head of his penis. It was a superficial tear, like the outer tissue was ripped. That went on for a few years until they researched having reconstructive surgery. In her case, the surgeon pulled some skin together from the inside, the entryway, and pulled it down to meet the location of the tear and seamed it together. Dr. Echenberg said that the surgery described by Bill is a vestibulectomy. The surgery eliminated the tearing problem, but the pain persisted. They even waited eight weeks after surgery to attempt intercourse, four weeks longer than recommended.

While they hoped the problem would be resolved, they understood that this Band-Aid surgery didn't get at the underlying problem, whatever it was. Once or twice a year Jackie used a thin dildo to test how she felt, but the pain was still too great.

In addition to the medical doctors, Bill and Jackie have seen five different types of therapists, from a psychiatrist to psychologist, social workers, and finally to a board-certified sex therapist. He said Jackie was never comfortable or willing to be self-revealing.

The truth of it for those of us who suffer is that while a psychological and emotional component exists, the pain is truly physical. It's caused by a myriad of neurological misfires that have entrenched themselves in our bodies, sometimes over decades. But with no diagnosis, there is no possibility of appropriate treatment. It's clearly a three-legged stool; we can't ignore the emotional and psychological, but without addressing the physical, one of two things happen: one, women feel crazy and misunderstood, as if they are to blame for the problem; and two, the emotional and psychological issues can't be healed without validating the physical. It's like an alcoholic trying to recover without putting down the drink. It's impossible.

I asked Bill if Jackie tried pelvic floor physical therapy, and he responded, "Forget it! She went and didn't like it. She wouldn't go back. My wife has an objection to being probed or touched."

They tried to watch erotic movies, but that backfired. Bill said that even if she was getting in the mood, seeing other people engaging in intercourse deflated her desire because, as he put it, "She's thinking 'it's unfair that that those woman can do it and I can't.' She'd get angry, even jealous."

For the next five years—from year 10 to 15 of their marriage—Jackie felt even more obligated to sexually satisfy her husband, even if she didn't want to do so. Fifteen years into the marriage, their sexual difficulties peaked. He described what would happen:

> She had not reached a point of pushing against me or blocking it with her muscles. My penis would slide in and then depending on how long she could stand it is how long I got to go before I pulled out. But as of today, I probably haven't ejaculated inside of her in 10 years.

PASSIONLESS SEX DESTROYS THEIR INTIMACY

Since then, sex for Bill and Jackie has primarily been comprised of mutual masturbation and oral sex. Bill told me it's become so repetitiously boring that he now has difficulty ejaculating at all, which tears him apart.

> She's gorgeous physically. When we're not in bed, she walks past me and I want to jump her bones. But in bed, she just wants to "service me," but not with any heart in

it or any sparkle in the eye, any romance, or any indulgence in the fantasy aspect. It's like having a podiatrist jerk you off.

The pain has removed Jackie's ability and desire to be sexy, essentially destroying a core part of her being. Beautiful on the outside, but terrified, angry, depressed, and empty on the inside. I suspect that because Jackie hurt from nearly the moment she lost her virginity, she associated sex with pain, so why would she want to engage in it? Never knowing the pleasure that others have enjoyed, she must have experienced deep grief.

PRESSURES INCREASE WITH FINANCIAL INSECURITY

Today, financial insecurity plagues the couple as well, which increases their tension. Despite an extremely successful career over three decades as a mid-level project manager, Bill had a spate of bad luck when the last two companies for whom he worked downsized. Over the past few years, it's taken him longer and longer to find a new position due to the emphasis on youthful energy and increasingly complex technology.

Bill is now a consultant, building on his storehouse of knowledge to give companies a conceptual edge. Still, it's not steady work, and five years of financial strain decreased his own self-esteem, leaving both he and Jackie with significant fear. It's also brought up anger and arguments about their finances. Bill said, "I think this situation has devalued me in her eyes. Her interest in me seems to have further waned with my unemployment as well."

INFIDELITY IS OFF THE TABLE

Bill insisted that he never cheated on Jackie. Fully devoted to her, he said, "I keep her on a pedestal, even under these conditions, and I'm always with her. I don't go out. I don't hang with friends. I don't have a card night. I don't go to titty bars. I don't drink. I don't smoke. I don't gamble. I love being at home with my wife, except for the sexual confrontations and frustrations that make me want to put my head through the wall."

So, what *has* kept Bill in the relationship for well over two decades? He said it's because they are best friends, plus he has an additional attachment that tears him apart:

> I think I'm totally addicted to her. It's like a drug addiction. But it's miserable to lie in bed next to a woman you want and can't have night after night. I'd stare at the ceiling, thinking, "I would just so love to roll over and feel her body next to mine." I'd like to make love to her. I want her to want me.

Bill and Jackie have discussed separation because they are increasingly living like two strangers. He lamented, "How do you live your entire lifetime and never truly enjoy your sexuality?"

Bill knows how hard it is for his wife to live with CPP, to be dismissed by doctor after doctor, to be told it's just in her head, to have surgery and find she's no better. He knows, as her partner, he must stand by her because he loves her. However, because he isn't the one with the physical pain, he's confused about how to find his way out of the emotional torture he endures and asks, "Is there a point beyond which a man has to move on or his own masculinity and self-image are destroyed? How do you go on with no intimacy?"

Acceptance is not easy for Bill at this point. He saw three therapists, hoping to find a positive solution, but instead, each therapist suggested his marriage was no longer the right fit. His confusion increased, as he explained, "I can't change my ethics, morals, or my friendship and loyalties to her. I just suffer every day. And I'll tell you what. I never, never, never dreamed that I'd be in my 30s, 40s, and my 50s, having to masturbate more than I have sex with my wife."

LIVING WITH CPP: SUSAN'S JOURNAL

When I finished editing Bill's interview, I felt a lot of anger for the mixed messages in it. One minute, Bill despaired about the couple's lack of intimacy; the next, he talked about their continuing attempts at sex and his wife's trying so hard to give him pleasure. He even mentioned her consistent ability to have an orgasm with him. Doesn't that count for something? Doesn't she get points for that?

Jackie continues to suffer to this day, the person without a diagnosis, the person without hope. In my opinion, it was his continued insistence on having intercourse that finally totally turned her off to sex completely.

Was Bill left unscathed in all this? No. He was as much a victim as she. But it was perplexing to me why I couldn't fully accept that or have more sympathy for him. I needed to figure this out.

First, I called a friend from college that I hadn't spoken with in nearly a year. We are close in that way we have with some people, as if, each time you do connect, it's like you are just continuing the last conversation. I called her because I remembered that, in her mid-40s, she'd been misdiagnosed with a sexually transmitted disease (STD) a few months into a significant relationship. The doctor never performed any tests on her, just made a decision from visual impression. The boyfriend did not have the STD. My friend underwent painful acid treatments that never helped and, she found out later, were not warranted. Obviously, intercourse was out of the picture.

Many months after severing her relationship with that doctor, she saw another gynecologist. By then, the symptoms had vanished on their own, so there was nothing to see except some scars from the acid. It turned out a test for this particular STD did exist. She took it, and the results were negative. Apparently, what she had was a severe bacterial infection. By then, unfortunately, her relationship had ended, too damaged to repair, so this good news came too late. As always, other issues contributed to the breakup. In this case, their respective life goals were too different, but my friend was convinced that had the STD episode not occurred, they would have worked through everything else. This was what particularly interested me.

Prior to her illness, her boyfriend wanted intercourse every day—without it, he felt something was fundamentally wrong in the relationship, as she explained:

> This was how he bonded with me. He felt it was the truest form of intimacy possible, a merging of our souls. Once I was diagnosed, it devastated him that we couldn't make love. Nothing else sexually was good enough. It wasn't that he wasn't there for me or wasn't supportive. It was that, without that connection, the intimacy was so much harder to achieve and maintain. Emotional, not just sexual. We knew, or hoped, that the physical symptoms would pass. But the strain on the relationship was too much.

My friend has had nearly a decade to analyze this situation to death. She firmly believes that men who aren't in love with their partners or are in it just for sex aren't particular about how they "get off." It's about the end game. The orgasm. But to men who love their women, it's about the ultimate connection. That's what makes them feel close, she concluded, "If intercourse is the way that a particular man doesn't feel alone in the world, feels it is the intimacy that keeps him with his partner, then without it, it's not the right relationship for him. Look, if I was with a guy and the only thing that really did it for him was anal sex, then he wouldn't be the right partner for me."

Well, that made some sense. But I was still confused. So I went to the ultimate authority on this matter, my husband, Jay. He, too, is one of those men who believes that, without intercourse, sex is essentially incomplete. Plus, he also feels that sex is about love-making, not just "doing it." He's accommodated to the nature of our new sex life in many ways, but the yearning has never left him.

Nothing else feels the same to him, not a hand, not even oral sex. Yes, we can have an orgasm together, but there is still a sense of incompleteness for him. He feels that since we're made for procreation (even though we're not making babies these days), that's the most natural act. Look at animals. It's just instinct.

So what about women, many (most?) of whom can't have an orgasm internally but have this magic button on the outside with double or triple the number of nerve endings of a penis? "Oh, well," Jay said, laughing, "that's God's little joke." Maybe that explained why it didn't bother me that intercourse was going the way of the dinosaur in our house.

So I pressed him for more information on why compromise sex wasn't good enough for most men. He said, "It's like driving a three-wheeled car. It'll get you there, but it's just not the same as a four-wheeled vehicle."

"What about a motorcycle," I asked my cycle-hugging husband, smugly one-upping him. "Or trikes?"

"Stop over analyzing this, Susan," he grumbled. "I have to get back to work."

WHAT REALLY MATTERS IN A RELATIONSHIP

Toward the end of my conversation with my friend, she said, "When women are in their 20s and 30s, sex really matters. Once we hit 40, we realize what we really want is a special someone to lay his head on the pillow next to us." That was definitely true for me.

As they age, some men also start losing their drive and/or potency. Maybe it's the universe's way of saying, "Hey, you aren't going to have any more kids, so you don't really need it anymore. After all, people used to die at 40." This may explain why my husband is not as freaked out as a younger man would be. He still wants it, but at age 65, he just doesn't have the youthful vigor he had at 40.

Forgetting, for a moment, about the little blue pill, this physical shift may help a man compromise in a relationship with a woman who has sexual pain. It's interesting that the term *erectile dysfunction* is applied to what may be a natural progression for men as they get older. Like wrinkles. But apparently a lot of guys feel compelled to take that little blue pill because they've bought into the idea that they should still be a bull at age 70.

POSTSCRIPT FROM BILL

About eight months after our interview, I heard from Bill again. He told me he and Jackie split up. He was living alone in a basement apartment about 200 miles from home. He said:

> Unfortunately, things went very sour. Because she could no longer bear the pressure or guilt to move forward with more professional help (medical or mental), she said I had to agree to NEVER, EVER bring up sex again . . . even the discussion of sex. She no longer had any interest or libido, and wanted to write off sex forever. It was her way to survive without the terrible guilt she carried.
>
> I had the choice of accepting a zero intimacy agreement or divorce! I'm not stupid. She was actually trying to help by giving me this out.
>
> It took me a full month to decide what my answer would be. You must understand that I still (to this very day) love her very much. However without sex, touching, affection, or hope of future success as bonded mates, I had to choose to leave. We

are in a mediated divorce as I write you today. We're doing everything in our power to remain friends for our good and the best interests of our children.

It's so hard to try to start over after 26 years with my wife. I'm heart-broken and love starved. But I could not see the rest of my life going the way she required. She quit/gave up and I had no solutions. I've supported her situation and always continued to hope that we would resolve or at least compromise enough to move forward.

I intend to try and find a new relationship that will give me my chance for a truly romantic and satisfying future. Romance is clearly not all I'm looking for; I want a best friend too!

AND A POST-POSTSCRIPT

Many weeks later, I received this email from Bill:

Jackie and I have reconciled! We stopped all work on our divorce! This is a beautiful thing! I learned over these last seven weeks that I couldn't live without her. She was constantly on my mind. I know I still love her deeply and feel she will always be my best friend. I'm preparing to move back home!

Nothing specific has been discussed regarding our future sex life. She and I have agreed that we miss each other unbearably and feel like we are without half of our bodies and minds. Since we never stopped loving each other, we felt it best if I just came home. New rules to be established later.

I pledged not to expect any sexual gestures from her and I agreed not to mention sex. . . . She now feels safe and won't carry the guilt of disappointing me. If and when she feels ready . . . . I'll leave it up to her.

While I was living in that awful basement, I realized that I missed her more than I missed sex. I also noticed that my interest in sex was rather low. Maybe it's my age now that I'm turning 58. I may have had unrealistic expectations of what my sex life would be with another women. I found out . . . and it wasn't all that it was cracked up to be!

I assessed my love for her and her kindness, intelligence, wisdom, loyalty, and nurturing nature, and decided I'd rather live with her than without her. Even if it means no sex. I do think she will feel safe enough that we could develop new affections for each other, like holding hands or snuggling up on the sofa . . . just nice, warm, and fuzzy stuff. Right now that's all I'll need.

Jackie and I believe that our two months apart allowed us to see both the good and bad in each other. We've drawn a line in the sand and are stepping over it into our new beginning. I pray that this will be the path to finding a happy way to live, love, and like each other again!

Wish us all the luck in the world! My heart has never been at such risk!

Perhaps love *does* conquer all. We'll see. As of this writing, that e-mail was the last I heard from Bill.

Chapter Seven

JENNIFER AND LISA: A SAME-SEX COUPLE'S STRUGGLE WITH SEXUAL PAIN

In working on *Secret Suffering*, I was surprised that out of hundreds of women who got in touch with me, no gay women responded to my calls for interviews. I felt uncomfortable that *Secret Suffering* would focus only on heterosexual relationships because chronic pelvic pain (CPP) has no sexual orientation. Any woman can experience vaginal pain (whether from penetration by a penis, a partner's fingers, tampon, diaphragm, or a vibrator), sexual pain in other areas (such as the clitoris, vulva, lower back, or stomach), and pelvic pain outside of the bedroom that lead to disrupting relationships in all areas of women's lives.

Fortunately, one of Dr. Echenberg's patients and her partner agreed to a written interview, for which I'm extremely grateful. Their inspiring, eloquent story testifies to the universal nature of sexual pain and its effect on both partners. Earlier, we read about Jennifer's journey to find a diagnosis from ages 15 to 25. In her teens, she was told her pain was ovarian in nature, thought mistakenly that endometriosis was the cause, and finally learned that she had vulvodynia, interstitial cystitis (IC), irritable bowel syndrome (IBS), and pelvic floor dysfunction. It is likely that trauma from competitive sports and sexual, physical, and emotional abuse as a child contributed to a build-up of the conditions that erupted.

In this part of Jennifer's story, we discover another side to the pain: how it affected her sexual life as an adult and her ability to experience emotional intimacy. At the age of 19, Jennifer became sexually active. Even during her first experience with a close male friend, Jennifer hurt so badly when he tried to penetrate her that she made him stop. "The pain felt like my vagina was tearing and went straight through to my lower back," she told me. "It was so bad, I couldn't think about anything else."

Jennifer tried to minimize her body's cries for help by convincing herself that all women experienced the level of pain she had during sex and during her menstrual cycles. She said:

> Doesn't everyone joke about "the morning after" when they feel a bit sore from having sex the night before? Doesn't every girl fight with a yeast infection now and then? I mean, why are there so many products out there for having a better sex life, fighting the occasional yeast infection, and relieving menstrual cramps and pain?
>
> This is how I viewed "my body's life." It had good and bad days and when it got cranky, it complained. I felt as if my body had an agenda all its own, leaving me in the dark most of the time. I couldn't understand how to read the simplest signals it sent me.

Within a short time, even oral sex was painful for Jennifer, especially involving the clitoris. In addition, her pelvic area hurt with any kind of penetration, even from a partner's finger. "There was a period of time when insertion was pleasurable," she explained. "But if her finger hit a certain spot, I had to ask my partner to stop. In some cases that was the end of any discussion, and often the relationship, for that matter."

Jennifer described the symptoms that had morphed from pain related to cycles and cysts into agonizing tentacles radiating into other parts of her body. "I felt a constant stabbing pain in my lower back and inner thighs," she explained. "It felt as if my pelvic muscles and tendons were grabbed by sandpaper hands and pulled and stretched. In addition, I had a pulsing pain throughout the pelvic area and lower back, up to my ribs and down to my knees. Any sexual penetration became impossible because of this pain."

She urinated between 10 and 12 times a day, suffered extreme nausea and headaches, and as a result, had little appetite. Jennifer said, "I couldn't wear anything tighter than soccer shorts or track pants—and no jeans." Her severe condition caused her to miss "countless days" of both school and work.

JENNIFER'S ROCKY ROAD TO LOVE

Jennifer met her life partner, Lisa, about seven years prior to this interview. Their relationship began as roommates after Jennifer, who had turned to drugs and alcohol to numb the physical and emotional pain, decided to clean up her life and "change people, places, and things." Lisa offered a safe haven and unconditional friendship. At first, despite their closeness as platonic friends, Jennifer didn't confide in Lisa about her condition, except to speak in general terms about her painful menstrual cycles. Four years after they met, Jennifer and Lisa fell in love. Jennifer explained:

> I thought Lisa and I would do very well sexually because we were so open to talking about everything right from the get-go. I felt more confident and comfortable in the first four days of our sexual relationship than I had in the entire span of other relationships. The fact that we truly felt connected spiritually allowed me to be much more at ease regarding sex. I felt respected, and Lisa treated me in a gentle and caring way from the first time we made love.

Lisa said:

> The evolution of our relationship was so natural and the respect so innate that even with our respective emotional baggage, when we first made love, it didn't occur to either of us to do anything other than listen to each other, both physically and emotionally. Ironically, because of my own issues, I was the one who became more guarded and withdrawn sexually as time went by.
>
> It was only after talking in depth and over a considerable length of time that the intimacy issues began to surface and be discussed openly.

It turned out that the secret Jennifer kept, once revealed, helped them both heal on emotional and spiritual levels. Once Lisa understood the depths of the pain Jennifer had suffered silently during sex, she said:

> My immediate reaction was horror that I could unknowingly hurt Jennifer. I was both mystified and keenly aware (due to my own issues) why she was hesitant to raise the topic. I don't remember any conversation about the future of our sex life. It was simply understood that we would take things as they came, and at Jennifer's pace.

Despite the fact that both women were healing, Jennifer admitted, "That didn't change our lives in some fairytale flash of hearts, clouds, and floating cherubs." In fact, shortly after beginning their romantic relationship, Jennifer became clinically depressed and lost all interest in sex. She couldn't deal with facing sexual pain on top of the emotional angst she suffered. Consequently, they had virtually no sexual contact for two years. But Lisa continued to love and support her.

Jennifer said the couple tried to compensate as best they could by "just curling up together and watching a movie, or playing games together." But she told me there was no denying that the lack of physical intimacy left an abyss between them and caused both to withdraw emotionally and physically. Jennifer at times thought the relationship would fall apart over it:

> I felt a huge amount of guilt because of my pain while having sex, as if I weren't a good enough partner, and because we didn't have sex for long periods. Lisa and I both view sex as not only a physical act but a spiritual connection, so it really was an issue when we went for months without having sex. She often said she missed making love and being close to me.

I also became very depressed and frustrated because I felt all the responsibility for sex was on me because Lisa said she would only respond to my requests to make love and not ask for sex. I was angry at her about this for a while, but mostly angry at myself for not being able to have a normal sex life with my partner.

Intimacy is far more than sex to Jennifer's partner. Lisa loves snuggling while watching a movie or reading with Jennifer. They'd developed a history together before they stopped having sex, which helped shore up the relationship. Lisa expressed her viewpoint:

We probably made love once every five to six months for a two-year span. For me, remembering how much we enjoyed just kissing and telling each other something new, or even just giggling together, can go a long way. This is certainly not to say that when our intimacy came to a standstill I was OK with that immediately. I wasn't.

However, I never pushed Jennifer in any way; instead, I withdrew emotionally and probably physically to a certain extent. Although I understood what was going on intellectually, I was frustrated.

THE JOURNEY TOWARD HEALING

Of her own journey toward healing, Jennifer said:

After I started to accept Lisa's love and allowed myself to love back without fear of negative repercussion, I slowly began to face and process the pain in my life. Before I could fully immerse myself in a loving relationship, I needed to find a harmony between the two parts of me that had been strangers to one another for so long. While I sought psychological help a few years ago, I realized that I had been on a journey to find the physical healing I needed for over 11 years.

After beginning to see Dr. Echenberg last year, she feels significantly improved. In addition, Jennifer is now in touch with her body and understands why the pain attacks her and where the pain comes from.

I'm happy to say I can now enjoy sex with my partner without any pain, which is wonderful. I can also differentiate regular aches and pains versus trigger points of pain. I'm able to point out spasms and better communicate where the pain radiates. In a relatively short time, I have had a life-changing experience.

Jennifer and Lisa have resumed their sex life. Now, during sex, she lets Lisa know right away when she's getting close to having pain during penetration and Lisa stops. Jennifer said, "When that happens, she'll change the amount of pressure she is using, where she's touching, and slow her movements down dramatically, or we'll have oral sex."

ADVICE FOR WOMEN WITH CPP FROM JENNIFER

Jennifer shares this advice for other women from what she's learned:

Break down your sexual pain symptoms into smaller, manageable pieces and work on each at a slow enough pace that you don't feel overwhelmed or burn out emotionally. If you're in a relationship, try talking about the pain in general terms and then introduce the individual symptoms. Talk about each at length, even if it seems too insignificant to discuss.

Make sure you cover *everything* because each little component of the sexual pain is important emotionally, spiritually, or physically, even if doesn't seem so at the time.

Spend a lot of time cultivating your relationship, dealing with the thoughts that "I should perform this way" or "I'm not good enough because I have sexual pain." Realize exactly how much pressure is put on you regarding sex: pressure from yourself, your partner, your friends, the media, etc. Know that sex isn't the be all and end all of relationships.

Make sure you are keeping tabs on your self-esteem, because it's very easy to lose it if you have sexual pain and are not actively attempting to talk about it, seeing a doctor for it, or providing some sort of outlet for all your emotions.

For the first time in my life, I can say I no longer feel I'm getting only a temporary fix or putting a band-aid over the problem. Instead, I'm truly taking the steps needed to become healthier and gain control over pain. I no longer feel that pain is so inextricably linked to my identity.

ADVICE FROM LISA FOR PARTNERS OF WOMEN WITH CPP

Lisa offered this conclusion about her experience as the partner of a woman who suffers:

Partners of women with pelvic and sexual pain need to have patience. Although the sexual aspect of a relationship is valid and important, it certainly isn't all encompassing.

It's vital to have empathy. Even if what your partner feels seems alien to you, everyone can find a personal experience to draw from where they needed unconditional love and support. Remember you are with this person because you fell in love with her.

Whether sexual pain enters your relationship after you've been together for a while or presents itself earlier on, she's still the same person. It's important to also realize that it's not a judgment upon you. Please show up as much as you can, physically, mentally, and emotionally. The biggest strain on a relationship comes with the loss of intimacy caused by both the emotional and physical pain. The longest 12 inches is from your head to your heart.

Chapter Eight

THE DILEMMA OF SINGLE WOMEN WITH CHRONIC PELVIC PAIN

I went through a period when I felt I wasn't loveable anymore, I was damaged goods, and that no man would want me. I felt lousy physically, mentally, emotionally. And it made me think I had no value.

—Marcie (interviewee)

So I tell men, "Before I start to get attached and this becomes an issue between us, tell me now if you can't deal with it and I'll just let you walk out the door and not worry about it hitting you in the ass on the way out."

—Pauline (interviewee)

For single or divorced women with sexual pain, dating becomes an even more daunting prospect than it is for the millions of unattached women without it. I spent a lot of years single—married first at age 34 and divorced at 40, then married again in my mid-40s.

I don't remember having much pain with intercourse until I was with my current husband for about a year and a half. This is not to say I never had problems with sex. I've already written about those so-called infections that dogged me and growing up with a constantly stinging urethra. I have fuzzy memories of experiencing so-called honeymoon cystitis when a boyfriend and I did it too many times. The agonizing pain the day after. Being told it was a bladder or vaginal infection. Dosed up with antibiotics too many times. Now, I wonder how often the doctors even did a culture before doling out the medication. I do remember the progression of vaginal burning, stinging urination, tight pants bothering me, and so on—all of which I experienced when I *wasn't* in a relationship.

I was one of the *very* lucky ones because my sex life began in the 1970s, right before the AIDS epidemic. It was sheer dumb luck that nothing bad happened to me. I didn't get AIDS, was not left with scars, not killed or raped by any of the men I brought home in desperate and confused attempts to find love, and have no warts or bugs or herpes lying dormant in my system, ready to spring up at an inopportune moment. But chronic sexual and pelvic pain is a progressive condition. Therefore, because I had symptoms even as a little girl, with stinging and burning down there, but wasn't diagnosed before my chronic pelvic pain (CPP) became so pervasive, here I am, at age 53, knowing that I'm lucky to have a good husband who will stand by my side because it's not very likely, with all this baggage, that I would find another.

Although I feel sad for young girls who are coming of age with such issues, I know there is more hope for them to get early treatment if we can educate them to recognize the symptoms as soon as they begin experiencing them and encourage them to find a knowledgeable doctor right away. Unfortunately, there are plenty of older women who already have CPP firmly locked in and have to face the world as single women, making tough decisions about dating and relationships.

A MARRIED WOMAN'S THOUGHTS ON BEING SINGLE WITH SEXUAL PAIN

Lauren's marriage has matured over decades. About it, she said, "There's a lot of love going on in a lot of different ways that are not sexually related. If you have that foundation, then the little things you do for each other during the day can take the edge off of other things you might feel you need to do sexually." However, if she found herself single, she had this to say:

It would be a whole different ball game. I don't think I'd want to get involved with anybody. He might make too many demands and I couldn't handle that. I need sexual release but I can do that myself.

I don't need to let somebody down, because the bedroom is all about performance—what I can do for you and what you can do for me. It just can't be negative. I don't want to hear a guy saying, with a disgusted tone of voice, "If you just tried harder, you could do it." If that were his take, it would make me feel bad for days. This attitude would overflow into all the other good areas of our life together.

I agree with Lauren. It's unimaginable to me that any man other than one with whom I've built some history would put up with my sexual pain issues.

WILL MARCIE FIND HER IDEAL MAN?

For Marcie, her problems began in 1989, in her late 30s. She was diagnosed with Lyme disease, fibromyalgia, and rheumatoid arthritis. She said, "I had

three bull's eye rings on my belly. Eventually, it began taking over my joints."
Her condition was discovered shortly after a car accident. She also had pelvic
and sexual pain, an ovarian cyst that was removed, and a diagnosis of interstitial cystitis.

At the time, Marcie was in a bad relationship and under a lot of stress. All
this, combined with her conditions, made intercourse impossible if she wasn't
relaxed. She said:

> When I feel stress, I clench my lower back and thighs. I had some pain on the right
> side of my vagina and my clitoris was sensitive to the point of pain. When I get
> upset, I'm not aware that I'm clenching so hard, but within a few hours, I start to feel
> the pulling in the clitoris. It's swollen and feels like a sharp needle going into it.

Marcie described her pain being on the right side only. Her theory is that
being right-handed meant that side of her body was stronger, which meant she
would clench harder on that side. Anything that rubbed against her with the
slightest pressure caused pain. She said, "It got to the point where I couldn't wear
pants or underwear. I had to cut little holes in my underwear and wear skirts."

Soon thereafter, she ended her relationship, which removed a lot of stress
surrounding sex. Ten years later, she hasn't had another sexual relationship. A
few years ago, she began seeing Dr. Echenberg. Because Marcie had not had
a sexual relationship in all this time and was careful to avoid any pressure on
her genital area, she was unaware of the pain simmering within her vagina
until she saw Dr. Echenberg. Once she started a course of bladder instillations
as part of her treatment, she realized that her pain was not only clitoral, but
within the vagina as well.

Today, at age 52, Marcie admits to being lonely but is afraid of entering into
a relationship, saying, "I'm hesitant and scared about this, but at the same time,
as I get older, I really don't want to be alone." She hopes to meet a man in his
40s, 50s, or 60s—a man she describes this way:

> I'm looking for someone who will be more concerned about personality and how
> we interact than the sex part. I'm hoping. I know that sex is important. But if I can
> satisfy a man in other ways, with oral sex or with manipulating or manually helping
> make it a wonderful experience for him, then he won't, well, I don't think, care—as
> long as I give him that release and enjoyment.
>
> Now, I'm not saying I wouldn't have intercourse at all. I'm just saying that if it's
> too sore, I'd tell him, "Hey, I have a problem." And make it more like a massage
> experience for both of us.

Ah yes, I wanted to tell Marcie, in an ideal world—the world in which you
didn't actually have to push him off of you or listen to the endless whining—
this might happen. But in the real world of most women with CPP who are
in a relationship, you're caught between knowing that to give in would mean

feeling agony and devising a plan to bring him to orgasm without intercourse. The complexity of creating this plan on the fly can be nearly as painful and exhausting as simply giving in.

At the time of our interview, Marcie confessed to having a crush on a man at work. While they're still at the flirting stage, she alternated between giddy anticipation and high anxiety. Her feelings came from years of living with the fear that sex will most likely hurt and not having had an intimate relationship within which to work through these issues for a decade. She further explained how she felt:

> Once you have a problem with sexual pain, it plays on your mind. It ups your stress. It just gets worse and worse and worse. You're not able to talk about it to anybody, you think you're all alone, and you don't know where to get help.
>
> I think there's still the possibility that I can find a relationship, if it's with an older man. And if I don't, I'm no worse off than I am now.
>
> But what I really want to know is this: Why can't they just make this go away?

PAULINE TELLS IT LIKE IT IS, UP FRONT

Earlier, we read about Pauline who put her foot down about not having painful sex and then divorced her insensitive husband. She has not remarried. Pauline was forthcoming about her dating philosophy, which can be summed up as preferring to keep the "dead elephant" *out* of the living room, rather than trying to move the beast later:

> Right after my divorce, I met a man online. I told him I had a problem before we started dating. When we were chatting online I said, "You seem pretty cool. Let me tell you this up front." And that's how I approach men: "I like you. You like me. Here's the catch."
>
> It's a fine line. After all, maybe someone who grew to care about you would be supportive. But putting that weight on someone before you develop a relationship may keep one from ever occurring. On the other hand, why waste time?

What happened after she told this new man about her sexual pain? During the nine months they went out, Pauline said he was accepting of her sexual limitations. However, they broke up for "personality reasons, not sex."

Pauline has had other men in her life since then, but it's been a rocky road, and she hasn't had a sexual relationship for nearly two years. Lots of women *without* sexual pain spend years searching for the right man. Although sexual pain is an impediment, let's face it, everyone brings a problem or two into a new relationship.

A few months ago, Pauline met a guy she really liked. As they grew to know each other, she shared her problem with him. The dialog between them went like this:

him: You know, I just don't really know if I can live without sex for the rest of my life.

her: I'm not asking you to live without sex for the rest of your life. I'm just telling you some nights I'll say, "No, get away." It's just one of those things, and if you can't deal with it, you need to let me know now because I don't want to put effort into this relationship if you can't deal with it.

him: Well, let me think about it.

her: If you've got to think about it, we're done.

Needless to say, this relationship didn't live to see another day. Most of her relationships over the past year have just been flings, dating for a month and they're done. "Nothing serious," she said, "No real sex."

LIVING WITH CPP: SUSAN'S JOURNAL

I was 30 to 60 pounds overweight for much of my adult life. It was hard to find a date, much less a boyfriend. I carried my pain on the outside and the inside. But even when I got thin, it was tough. My personal guesstimate is that it's difficult for 99 percent of women to find the right man, but the added layer of sexual pain makes it even more challenging to exude the allure that attracts a man. It takes guts to spit out the painful truth because it's not only embarrassing, but downright humiliating, especially knowing that the response may not be the one we want to hear. But I'm with Pauline. I'd rather get it out of the way up front to clear out the dead weight.

Chapter Nine

OUR RELATIONSHIPS OUTSIDE THE BEDROOM

I know it sounds funny, but I missed two of the key scenes of a movie I really wanted
to see last week because I had to pee twice in 45 minutes. I tried to ignore the persistent pressure in my bladder, telling myself, "Just a few more minutes." But when the
pressure turned to pain, there was no choice.

—Survey respondent

I live with severe vaginal burning. Each day, I suffer through work, then come home
and sit on a cold beer bottle. It's like heaven. I keep two beer bottles in the fridge.

—Lydia (interviewee)

My grandmother died at the end of December and I had to sing at the funeral. I
was having a hard time making it through the songs. And that devastated me because I was supposed to be paying respect to my grandmother and I couldn't even
do that without having to run up and down the steps every 10 seconds to go to the
bathroom.

—Kat (interviewee)

Our illness spills outside of the bedroom. Just going through life presents
exhausting challenges. Sometimes we have to say no to food or events that
we know will be too hard to manage. For instance, I am loathe to take a long
car ride with anyone in a hurry because I know that it's possible I'll be stopping every hour. When traveling, I go to the bathroom even more than I do
at home. I think the stress of *worrying* about going to the bathroom actually
increases my urgency. Just a charming little quirk, I guess.

Some women have to change jobs. Some women can't stand too long or sit
too long. Others are so ill from chronic pelvic pain (CPP) they need to take a

leave of absence, which leaves them financially strapped and more stressed out. Others have to confide in coworkers to cover up, having to sneak out for frequent doctor's visits. Getting through each day is sometimes more challenging than facing sex with a partner.

This chapter describes the devastation wrought by the demon of CPP on the other significant others in our lives: our families, friends, coworkers, and/ or educators and classmates. There are many complicated facets to this issue. We do our best to function in our environment, shoving the pain down to the best of our ability in order to maintain our responsibilities. This denial often makes us feel worse physically and takes a huge toll because we feel like we have to hide our suffering while pretending nothing is wrong. We don't want to be a burden, and for some of us, we don't want to put our jobs in jeopardy if we call in sick one too many times.

In addition, we may feel embarrassed and humiliated because we can't join our family or friends in activities we'd love to do but may cause us problems, such as bicycling, long hikes, going out to eat, taking a vacation, and so forth. Unfortunately, because there are rarely outward indications of our illness, when we do talk about the problem, some people look at us like we're from Mars, or worse, think we are feigning some smoke and mirrors illness.

As for our immediate family, if we become debilitated to the point where the pain shows no matter what, supportive adults and children alike are distraught watching us feel so miserable, standing by helplessly, and desperately wanting to make it better. This brings up one of the core issues psychologists in the field work on: helping the patient deal with the family's attitude toward him or her. According to Dr. Lyndsay Elliot, clinical psychologist, the attitude of the patient's family has a strong impact on her condition. "Being supportive, encouraging, and patient is essential. It's harmful, obviously, if there's any shaming going on or distancing from the family members. Making fun of them or teasing—those kinds of things can be difficult."

LOIS'S FAMILY LIFE

Lois's son and daughter are 32 and 29 and are very aware of her condition (vulvodynia, vulvar vestibulitis, and interstitial cystitis) and highly supportive. She said, "They know that if I stand when we're together, I'm just in pain and have to get up off my bottom." She described how she explained her condition to them:

I said I have a nerve problem down in the private area. I told them it's like a blow torch and like someone has grabbed it with pliers and twisted and won't let go.

I explained that the pain is excruciating and makes me have to get up and move around while I'm talking to them. They've just lived with it since 1994 . . . that's a long time. I have very understanding and compassionate children.

Lois's children watch to make sure their mom doesn't overdo it, but even after all these years struggling with pain, Lois is tenacious and her high energy level still simmers beneath the surface, wanting to come out fighting. She said that her children will yell at her if she does too much. "I try to be the person that I used to be. I'll do something and then the pain comes back. So, for instance, when I get a little frisky with the grandkids, they'll say, 'Mom, don't pick her up. Don't do this. Don't do that.' They say it because they know what's going to happen."

She also belongs to a hobby club that meets weekly. However, she cannot take on an active role, such as becoming an officer, because of her condition. Overall, she loves the club, but it's become a nightmare to appear normal. She said:

> The pain is so great when I'm sitting there that a lot of times I can't focus on what they're saying and people tend to think that I'm snobbish. But meanwhile, I'm only trying to get control of my life in a social situation.
>
> So I end up putting on a semi-smile, but inside I'm not listening to them because I'm trying to deal with the pain that's fired up. Most people don't know that about me because I tend to hide my pain. I don't go around telling everyone about it because no one wants to hear it. Like you said, it's the secret pain that nobody talks about.

Lois finds that her illness interferes with even the most basic decisions. This pain has ruled her life in so many small ways that most people would find unimaginable, even down to the choice of a family car. "I even have to pick out the car we buy to be sure I can sit on the seat," she said, a bit choked up. "My husband really wanted a Cadillac, but I made him buy the Buick because the seat was less irritating."

JANE'S FAMILY LIFE

As previously stated, Jane was diagnosed with vulvar vestibulitis, painful bladder syndrome (PBS), and pelvic floor dysfunction. Her parents have tried to be helpful, but she said, "They just don't get what this is or how I feel or how it affects me. My Mom keeps telling me, 'Well, you just need to do a little more every day, then you'll feel better again and you'll be stronger.' And I tell her that I'm not recovering from a virus. I have a chronic incurable illness."

Jane told me that a lot of the people with whom she's communicated online have severed relationships with parents and extended families due to their lack of understanding. She said, "You know, even for people who aren't married, it takes a toll on the family. When you get a chronic disease, it doesn't just happen to you, it happens to your whole family."

Jane was going through a flare-up when we spoke, but she told me that the medication she takes makes it bearable, as does lying in bed with a heating pad. Without those things, she said, "I'd probably be screaming and lying on the floor or would have killed myself by this point. But I have a daughter and that's the one thing that has really kept me holding on." Even at the age of seven, her daughter understood that she was ill. Jane said, "She knew Mommy was in the hospital or Mommy was in bed or Mommy was unable to drive because of medication."

When her daughter was nine, she explained to her what was wrong and that there wasn't a cure for it but there were good treatments:

> I told her that I had pain in my vagina, in my bladder, and in the sides of my pelvis. I showed her where that was. I explained that the pain was very bad and I had to take strong medication. She's extremely intelligent and I think she understood.

That same year, the mother of one of her daughter's classmates died, and her daughter's anxiety about Jane's condition escalated. She jumped in to reassure her, saying, "I want you to know that we're not keeping anything from you. Everything we told you is everything we know and I'm not going to die from this. I'll probably have times where I'll be better and times I may get worse again. But I'm always going to be here for you."

In the summer, she used to coach her daughter's swim team. Together, they'd play around in the water, doing flips and handstands. But when the pain became so severe that she could no longer share their summer fun, she and her daughter had to become resourceful to maintain their closeness. Even though Jane and her daughter have worked out ways to be together, she feels a lot of guilt about her inability to be active with her. "During the school year, she comes up and does her homework with me. We'll both prop ourselves up on cushions in my bed and she'll do her homework right next to me. She can look up and talk to me and I can help her. That's nice quality time. I bought her some board games that we can do together. But it's not the same."

Her daughter is now 12. Over the years, she has had mixed reactions. According to Jane, she's sometimes irritated about her mother's limitations, but for the most part, she expresses great compassion and concern. Her daughter has taken on a lot of household responsibilities, such as doing the laundry and cooking. It tears at Jane's heart that she cannot be the mother she once was and that her condition has forced her daughter into an adult role that she shouldn't have to take on at such a young age. She described a recent incident:

> I was upstairs in bed. It was right after school and my daughter was down in the kitchen. Suddenly, I heard her sobbing. I would like to say that I ran down the stairs, but basically, I hobbled down as quickly as I could.
>
> It turned out that she had slammed her head into the handle of the microwave. I held her and comforted her and told her that it would feel better soon.

She said, "I'm so sorry, mommy, because you had to come down when it hurts you to do that, and you had to get out of bed when you were resting, and you need rest, and I'm so sorry that I made that happen to you."

I felt so awful. She doesn't even feel like she has a right to be mothered anymore and she's only in sixth grade. I just kept telling her "I'm the Mom. That's my job."

Jane ended her story by saying, "Chronic pelvic pain is a tremendous blow to your self-esteem and incredibly hard on one's psyche. I think depression is inevitable and we all have it to some degree or another, and it inevitably plays havoc with your family relationships."

BALANCING WORK AND PELVIC PAIN

Managing one's workload and keeping employers happy can sometimes be daunting because many women with sexual pain often need significant time off for doctor appointments, physical therapy, and just plain feeling ill. This is an especially difficult tightrope to walk with a chronic condition the patient doesn't wear on the outside. To be blunt, most women with pelvic pain don't look sick. So sometimes, coworkers and management may be less than sympathetic.

Valerie's Lack of Support at Work

Valerie, an ad agency marketing director, told me about a work incident that enraged her:

Somebody overheard one higher up person in our company say to another that she wasn't really buying into everything about my illness. I never confronted her on it because the person who told me didn't want her to know they overheard her say that, but I was livid. That woman had no idea what kind of treatments I've been going through. She thinks I'm just trying to get pregnant, I guess, going for fertility treatments or something.

Jane Loses Her Career to This Illness

Jane was a high school English teacher. The lead-up to leaving her job was emblazoned in her memory. Her CPP started simply enough; she used one tampon on vacation a week before school started and experienced severe vaginal burning by that evening, which never let up.

Her worsening condition caused her concentration to decrease. More stress was added to her already weakened immune system with the drawn-out death of her uncle. She said she began making an increasing number of mistakes due to pain and fatigue. When she gave incorrect standardized tests to three classes, she was strongly encouraged to take a leave of absence by her angry boss. Teaching was everything to Jane. She didn't want to leave her students, but eventually, she not only took the leave, but ended up quitting entirely.

Because she cannot walk too far, she got a handicapped parking placard. But, she said, "When I use it and get out of the car, people look at me like there's nothing wrong with me. I think they think I'm cheating."

She's now getting state disability and has applied for Social Security disability because she's so afraid that even if she has a remission from her illness, she'll never know when it will return. And thus, a much-needed teacher who cares had to step down due to an illness that doesn't care.

LIVING WITH CPP: SUSAN'S JOURNAL

One of my symptoms, as you probably know by now, is a chronic need to pee. I'd like to be more politically correct, but I'm just not going to write urinate 200 times. And now that I drink a lot more water, I need to pee even more, but thankfully, it rarely burns and stings like it used to in the past.

My son, Sam, plays the clarinet in the high school marching band. They often compete quite a distance away. Trying to be an involved parent, I decided to be a chaperone and go on the bus with the band to one of their competitions, a four-hour drive to Inverness, Florida.

Prior to the trip, Sam informed me numerous times that going to the bathroom on the bus was not allowed. That seemed ludicrous at the time. But when I showed up at 6 A.M. on the morning of the trip, I had a kernel of anxiety balling up in my stomach, so I blithely asked two of the in-charge parents about this obviously ridiculous edict. My worst fear was realized. "Oh, no," they blurted out in unison, looking horrified. "Once that toilet is flushed, even if it's number one, it's too awful. The stench! Oh, no, you just can't."

Now, I was stuck. My anxiety sprouted from a kernel into a bowl of expanding popcorn terror. I forced myself to pee three times before boarding and was on the verge of a panic attack the whole trip up. I was afraid to drink water. They stopped twice, which, luckily, was enough.

Once we arrived, I discovered the bathroom was a five-minute walk from the stadium. Three stalls, 10 bands, hundreds of girls and dozens of female chaperones. I was smart—after the first time. I went to wait in line long before I felt even the twinkling of an urge. I got a lot of exercise that day.

Upon boarding the bus to go home (at midnight), the in-charge mom announced that we would drive straight through on the return trip. My panic overcame my embarrassment. "*No!* I, uh, no, we have to make a bathroom stop," I shrieked. The entire busload of teenagers stared at me. I tried to manage a weak grin and just said, "Menopause," with a shrug. I thought, the 40-something in-charge mom would understand that, but she just looked at me with annoyance. I knew it made no sense; it was just the best I could do at the time.

But a miracle happened. We stopped. We peed. We arrived safely home.

And, in the end, the trip was worth all the anxiety because my son was actually glad that I was there. He didn't say it, but his demeanor showed it. He joked with me right in front of his friends, let me take pictures, and, once in a while, I even detected a smile when he glanced my way.

They didn't win the competition, but they gave it their best effort. And maybe I can't win the war against my pelvic pain, but I can put up a hell of a fight to ensure I don't miss out on the important moments in my son's life.

Chapter Ten

LISTENING TO OUR DAUGHTERS

I was a cheerleader for nine years. You're not meant to be thrown around like I was. I really took a lot of abuse. You fall on the floor or you're falling and they're grabbing you by your wrists and you're hanging there. It's just not good. If I could, I would take back those nine years of cheerleading because it wasn't worth it.

—Tiffany, a college senior

The young female athlete who also has increasing irritating symptoms of bladder, lower bowel, and early teen menstrual pain, may eventually see a number of different specialists, but until now, it has been rare for any of these professionals to look at the whole picture and have the knowledge it takes to predict that this complex of symptoms and activities may later take such a huge toll on these young women's lives. Pediatricians, family physicians, athletic trainers, coaches, parents, and teachers alike all should have some awareness that these problems are common and know the signs, so preventative measures and appropriate treatments could be established before years of pain and suffering occur.

—Dr. Robert J. Echenberg

I was diagnosed with vulvodynia when I was 20, but I know I had it much longer than that. My family physician had no idea that vulvodynia was a condition and even went so far as to tell me that the pain was all in my head.

—A patient of Dr. Echenberg

There are a lot of things that you can fix. If someone has severe endometriosis and interstitial cystitis, for example, you identify every one of the problems and treat every one of the problems. You can usually fix those patients, if you catch them early.

If you catch them too late, the pain centralizes, and then it's more a matter of control than it is a cure.

—The late Dr. C. Paul Perry

Clarissa is 23 years old and has already had a hysterectomy. As she recounted her story, I saw a woman who grew up fast because of her determination in the face of little parental support to find help for her solitary pain. She said:

> For me it started with long periods and heavy bleeding when I was 13. The pain just progressed from there, from about seven days to two weeks at a time.
> My pain stays in my left quadrant and it's about the size of a softball. It feels like somebody is stabbing me. It's always there. If I'm stressing out and having intercourse, the pain just spreads. It spreads to my back and into my legs, and now everywhere, so it's really strange.

I thought about the prevalence of pelvic pain in young girls. Many women don't realize until they've found a proper medical provider who thoroughly questions them about their medical history that they've had their symptoms for years, often beginning as a teenager. For a young woman on the brink of blossoming sexually and entering into intimate relationships, beginning this phase of her life equating sex with pain is tragic.

When I asked Clarissa about her experience with doctors throughout the 10 years prior to our interview, she related a story no different than many I'd heard before, saying, "Most doctors didn't believe me, or if they believed me they were trying to put me on injections. I've been on tons of birth control and they put me on Lupron injections to try to stop my periods, but that didn't work."

Clarissa's parents divorced when she was young. Many women with chronic pelvic pain (CPP) were sexually abused at some point in their lives. Clarissa is one of these victims. However, she declined to discuss this subject, though she told me she had gone to therapy to deal with the wreckage of the experience.

When she was 13, she tried to tell her mother about the pain. She said:

> My mom didn't believe me. She didn't believe that I had even started getting my period so it was an awkward situation. I would tell her that I had really, really bad cramps and she would say, "Oh, that's normal." She didn't even take me to the gynecologist until I was 16 and I said there's something going on; I need to go.

Clarissa's mom died from a freak accident shortly thereafter. She was riding a bicycle and a truck mirror hit the back of her head. I'm sure that such a thing adds so much stress to an already pain-filled body. My own mom died of cancer after a six-year battle when I was in my mid-20s. To this day, I know that an irreversible toll was taken on my body, mind, and spirit. Instantaneous, unexpected death, however, makes a mark of abandonment that is profoundly shocking in its suddenness.

HER RELATIONSHIP WITH HER HUSBAND

Clarissa met Mitch when she was 18. At the age of 19, they began having sex. Now, Mitch and Clarissa have sex twice a week. She told me it hurt from the first time.

> It felt like there was something stuck in there, exploding from the inside out, stabbing on the top usually. I just thought, "Oh well, it's just because it's your first time having sex; this is what happens."

Clarissa kept having sex (intercourse) despite the pain. She'd just grit her teeth and bear it. Even now, years later, nothing much has changed. She said, "I don't want him to feel like, you know, denied."

Although Clarissa doesn't make Mitch stop, she will speak up. She told me, "Sometimes I'll say, 'I don't like it this way' or 'my hips hurt' so he'll change positions, but most of the time I'll just lay there, grin and bear it and be like 'ok, I hope you're done soon.' Usually I lay on my belly and I have my right leg out and he straddles my left leg. And that usually feels OK."

When asked if she has other types of sexual activity, she said, "Most of the time, it leads to intercourse. We have toys, but we don't really use them because they hurt me too. I help him and stuff, but he just still likes intercourse. He feels that it's more intimate, more like giving a piece of yourself. He says, 'Oh, I have to have it inside' and I'm like 'whatever.' Some days I have resentment and wish he'd just go away."

Clarissa has never experienced an orgasm. She's read a number of books to help her understand, but she still finds no pleasure in sex. She said, "It's usually just pain. And sometimes I'll get a little pleasure like 'Oh that feels nice' but then I usually pay for it afterward. It hurts worse afterwards. It just feels like . . . I'm going to die!"

Most telling about this youthful relationship was her feeling that Mitch doesn't understand enough to be sufficiently compassionate. When it comes to sex, she said, "He'll say, 'either don't tell me it hurts, or just tell me not to do it.' But I can't say that. I think it's because of the way I was brought up. You don't say no."

GOING TO EXTREME MEASURES

In 2006, at the age of 21, Clarissa saw an OB/GYN who couldn't figure out why she continued having pelvic pain. The doctor said she could have laser treatments and they could burn the inside of the uterus, but that it probably wouldn't work for the pain. So she had another laparoscopy and then, when multiple doctors still couldn't figure out what was wrong with her, they suggested a hysterectomy. And after the hysterectomy? She said, "I still had the pain."

Clarissa was finally referred to the doctor who diagnosed and treated her for painful bladder syndrome/interstitial cystitis (PBS/IC), pudendal neuralgia, and pelvic floor dysfunction. It turned out that she'd had excessive bladder urgency and frequency along with her pain the entire time, and no one paid attention to, or even asked about, those symptoms.

MANAGING CPP

While her physical relief has been intermittent, on an emotional level, Clarissa said that seeing a doctor who finally diagnosed her, continues to work with her, and believes her has made a big difference in how she feels about her life.

The day I interviewed Clarissa, the day she felt her best because she just had a pudendal block, was still not a day that was pain-free. "It's burning," she said, "but it's not as bad. I can deal with a little burning." So she plans to have sex with Mitch today, which she considers a good day.

Postscript

I heard from Clarissa six months after our interview. She and Mitch were separated and filing for divorce.

LIVING WITH CPP: SUSAN'S JOURNAL

One of the most important lessons from Clarissa's story for me is that it's so important to talk about sex with our daughters. We need to take our daughters seriously and believe them when they tell us they're in pain (and if they tell us they've been abused).

The world and the media push the young into sexual relationships so early. There's really a small window of time to help them ride the fine line of conscience, consciousness, and hormones. Our daughters need to feel safe to talk about the changes in their bodies as they mature.

I remember when I was 11, I was in the tub when there was a flush of blood. I dried off with panic in my heart and raced into my mother's room, where she was talking to her best friend on the phone. I blurted out that there was blood. Her reaction surprised me. She had a tone of near delight as she told her friend that I just got my period. Together, she and I figured out how to place that rubber contraption around my waist and put that pad in. (These were the days well before mini-pads). Though I'd read books, it was still terrifying to experience. I was lucky to have a parent who at least gave me a bit of guidance, but the vaginal/urethral stinging I experienced from age six or seven went without diagnosis until adulthood. All I remember of that is sitting in lots of hot baths to soothe the pain.

If my mother took me to the doctor for this condition at all, clearly she was satisfied with an answer that didn't solve the problem. It wasn't that she didn't love me; she loved me dearly. But if the doctor insisted, "it was nothing," in those days, no one argued with medical authorities because they "knew best."

For me and many other women, it took years in adulthood to figure out that the pain was not normal and to advocate for ourselves. However, if parents become educated and keep the lines of communication open, if they make it safe for young girls to let parents know if there is anything that doesn't seem right, they have an opportunity to quell their fears and find early answers.

Parents have an obligation to believe their daughters when they say it hurts. You must be their advocate to demand the help they deserve so they don't feel abandoned and grow up, grow old, with pain they think is normal or imagined.

By loving our daughters enough to listen and find them the appropriate medical help before the acute turns into chronic pain, we will pave the way to grow girls into women who have a voice to say no to doctors who won't listen, no to painful sex, no to painful relationships, and yes to self-confidence as they walk through life.

In Dr. Echenberg's Words

A number of young women barely out of their teens have suffered outrageous indignities at the hands of the medical profession. Some of these girls have been put through needless surgeries such as multiple laparoscopies, removal of ovaries, and even hysterectomies, as well as potent hormonal and pain suppressants that are often not warranted by their symptoms. Clarissa's story is especially tragic because of her young age. In our practice regarding chronic pelvic pain, we see many young women who have already been through the mill, like Clarissa.

Clarissa was diagnosed and treated for PBS/IC, which may well have been the main source or trigger for her chronic pelvic and sexual pain from a very early age. I have learned that women with PBS/IC have a considerably higher chance of having a hysterectomy than the average woman without bladder symptoms.

Hysterectomy, or any surgery, for that matter, is not the treatment for PBS/IC and should always be a last resort in any case for young women. It clearly wasn't the "fix" for Clarissa's chronic pain. The bottom line with a great majority of CPP patients is that they've had symptoms for years, even decades, that commonly began in childhood or adolescence and were never considered to be related to one another. And that's a tragedy.

Clarissa's case is not unique. So many of our patients are very young. Of course, we are most pleased when we encounter patients earlier in the course of their pain issues, but too frequently, their symptoms are already quite severe even in their teens or early 20s. As a doctor who has seen women at various ages who have often been subjected to years of disappointing and unsuccessful treatments for their pelvic pain, and whose relationships have suffered immensely because of chronic sexual pain, it has become glaringly obvious that these women needed to be diagnosed, treated, and stabilized at a much younger age.

COMPETITIVE SPORTS CAN START THE PELVIC PAIN CYCLE IN YOUNGER PATIENTS

According to Dr. Echenberg, "Typically women under age 35 or 40 have had histories of many more pelvic physical injuries than those who are older." He said that many such patients were more heavily involved in sports and other physically demanding activities than older women. Long-term participation in such activities as cycling, gymnastics, cheerleading, track and field, soccer, hockey, softball, dance, and horseback riding could all trigger future CPP.

Encouraging young women to be highly competitive in sports throughout their entire grade school, middle school, and high school years has become the norm over the past 20 years. Girls are worked hard—often, too hard. According to Dr. Echenberg, "The young body is not meant to be pushed to these limits."

Tiffany, a college senior and former cheerleader, said that when she fell, coaches never gave her any time to recover. "They said, 'Try again. Get back on the horse, Tiffany. We're gonna try this one again.' There was never a time out."

Samantha, a recent college graduate and patient of Dr. Echenberg, said, "I played competitive volleyball most of my life, which meant a lot of crashing onto the hard wood floor." She played straight through her junior year in college after four knee surgeries, a head injury that almost killed her, and numerous laparoscopic surgeries. She said, "You just keep playing. You never stop. You're taught to do that. Your coaches encourage that. It's your main goal because they expect you to be there the next day."

Samantha said that her coaches had her playing on the volleyball court after having knee surgery. She said, "I was literally on the court, having my knee drained three or four times, bleeding on the court, and my coach said, 'Man up and play.' I said to myself, 'What the hell am I doing?' I took off my jersey and never went back."

In Dr. Echenberg's Words

Michael Sokolove recently wrote a book titled *Warrior Girls—Protecting Our Daughters against the Injury Epidemic in Women's Sports.*[1] Sokolove is an investigative reporter from the *New York Times Sunday Magazine* who spent several years researching this issue. In his book, he talks about the likelihood of knee injuries, concussions, low back and hip injuries, and so forth, from these sports activities. I was greatly interested in his book because so many of our young patients have similar histories, and so many of these athletically inclined women have unfortunately even learned, as adults, how to have sex through the pain.

Sports programs appear to be deficient in recognizing the need for gender differences in the training of these young athletes. Sokolove also brings up the fact that young women are more bonded in their team relationships in sports than are young men, and consequently, the girls are more likely to play through the pain so as not to let down their teammates.

The tragic stories of young women who develop sexual/pelvic pain are at least partially preventable. In retrospect, we see that many triggers of pelvic and sexual pain began at quite a young age. These complexes of disorders and symptoms should never be written off as just plain old growing pains or normal emotional adjustments to their blossoming young bodies. These problems remain under the radar mostly because the individual, her family, and even health care professionals and trainers never link many of these factors together.

For most young female athletes, future pelvic and sexual pain problems will not be a consequence. However, we should be particularly aware that if our daughters are at risk of ongoing athletic injuries, and also are exhibiting increasingly painful menstrual, bladder, or bowel disorders, we should be cognizant that these young women are at higher risk. Often their entire passion is the sport to which they are devoting so much time and energy to master. While competition is a key component of sports, the health of our daughters is paramount.

Ironically, we are intent on curbing juvenile obesity and getting our young people more active and away from their sedentary lives of computer games and texting. Although those goals are high priority, we must still be cognizant of the cumulative injuries and functional disorders that our young women are experiencing and the potential for future pelvic pain and sexual dysfunctions.

LIVING WITH CPP: SUSAN'S JOURNAL

Dr. Echenberg has made it clear that we need to be more vigilant about protecting our daughters. We must educate ourselves and our daughters so they aren't afraid to let us know when they hurt. Coaches and trainers must cooperate with parents to ensure their daughters aren't left with a legacy of debilitating chronic pelvic pain that may destroy their lives, relationships, and even their ability to bear children after their school sports careers are over. There is no prize more precious than the health of our children and no win more important than the quality of life that follows the final big game.

But What About the Role of Our Sons in All This?

My son Sam is 18. Though he's the love of my life, being 18 means that he's a little bit (ok, completely) self-centered. Therefore, he has not been terribly compassionate about my condition. In fact, unless I can transport him, feed him, or give him money, nothing about my life is of particular interest to him right now.

He's thoroughly enmeshed with his (first) girlfriend, so I imagine he's facing his own sexuality (though I try to pretend otherwise for my own sanity). Before the girlfriend, he was horrified at the mention of my "unmentionables," as he called my pelvic pain, and practically put his hands on his ears, going "la la la la la" like a five-year-old, whenever I even mentioned it or the book.

Now, however, he seems rather nonplussed about it, though still pretty much disinterested. I'm hoping against hope that it's just because I've continued talking to him about it despite his protests, rather than his own sexual experience jading him.

Be that as it may, the most important point I've impressed upon him throughout my work on *Secret Suffering* is the prevalence of pelvic pain in young girls. He must realize that this isn't just an old lady problem. With estimates ranging from 12 to 39 percent of reproductive aged (teens through menopause) women suffering from pelvic pain at some point in their lives, it's just as important for our young men to become educated about pelvic and sexual pain as our young women.[2]

It's clear to me that our sons need to grow up with a strong sense of what commitment means, even in the face of hardship. There are no guarantees for any of us that we will remain healthy. We have classes in math, science, music, and economics. How about required courses in how to develop healthy relationships and the importance of loyalty and commitment despite adversity?

Relationships are difficult to begin with, and struggles are inevitable. But as Sam walks through life and love, I want him to be the kind of man who will understand and stand by his woman if a condition such as chronic sexual pain is the card they are dealt together.

Chapter Eleven

LORI: A YOUNG WOMAN OF FAITH

Twenty-four-year-old Lori is quite thin and lovely, with long blonde hair and big blue eyes. She's also a devout Christian who struggles with chronic pelvic pain. She doesn't believe in sex before marriage, but for a young woman wanting to experience a full life with a partner, the pain she experiences even now, along with the anticipated pain that sex will bring, looms large in making her decision about whether to even embark on a relationship. This young woman contacted me and allowed me to interview her.

Secret Suffering takes no position on any religion or faith. I, myself, am Jewish, and clearly, our common condition overwhelms any particular belief. However, I found Lori's point of view fascinating and relevant to any discussion of sexual and pelvic pain. It is only natural that a woman already experiencing chronic pelvic pain (CPP) symptoms (diagnosed or not) who has not yet engaged in sexual activity inevitably approaches intimacy with trepidation, an important aspect of sexual pain to explore. Further, how women of faith spiritually cope with this illness is yet another important point of view to present.

In her first letter to me, Lori explained how the pain is intertwined with her strong love for and faith in God. She said, "As incompatible as these two things may seem in common Christian beliefs, it's a daily fact for me. I find that true Christians believe, as I do, that God doesn't promise a life free from suffering; he simply promises a life free from boundaries from Him."

Gastrointestinal issues are considered a component of pelvic pain, and Lori's most intense symptoms are in her lower bowel. Through our conversation, I discovered she also experiences vaginal pain, but since she's never been sexually active, she's unaware of that discomfort unless an object is inserted, such as a tampon or a gynecological probe during an exam. It's highly likely that if she marries, her CPP will erupt in her sex life, a fear that haunts her.

WATCHING HER MOTHER'S STRUGGLE WITH INTERSTITIAL CYSTITIS

Lori understood the implications of a chronic pelvic pain condition because her mother began having pelvic floor issues and symptoms of interstitial cystitis (IC) 5 years into her marriage, about 25 years ago, when little was known about these conditions.

Therefore, Lori had grown up watching her mother and father deal with this difficult situation. She witnessed her father distraught at seeing the woman he loved in so much pain over the years, yet based on their experiences with the medical community and the treatments that only worsened her mother's condition, her parents felt helpless. She said, "Both of them were just stuck suffering."

ODE TO THE PAIN

I felt it was important to present Lori's story, both because she is a young, celibate woman, as well as the fact that the CPP symptoms of which she is most keenly aware are primarily related to gastrointestinal issues. I think many women don't realize that their stomach problems, such as those diagnosed as irritable bowel syndrome (IBS), are also manifestations of CPP and pelvic floor dysfunction. Lori can precisely describe the pain:

> There is a swelling pain, where I feel like an overfilled water balloon that longs to burst. I feel my skin stretch and my insides expand. This usually happens after I have eaten something unusual, but it isn't necessarily associated with how much I eat. This full feeling would be reasonable if I was gluttonous, but I tend to eat meager portions.
>
> A sharp pain on my left side takes my breath away. When I walk, the feeling worsens. Sometimes it feels like someone has taken a red-hot poker and jabbed it into my side. Other times I feel like someone has taken a knife and cut me in two.
>
> One of the worst sensations is a thrashing pain that feels like a boxing champion is beating my stomach into a bloody pulp. It leaves my stomach in knots. I also get a spiky pain, where I feel like I've swallowed a sea urchin and the spikes are grating away my insides. If I bend, the spikes feel sharper.
>
> Finally, I feel like a creature lives inside of me, gnawing at my insides, and won't leave. Mentally, this is one of the hardest feelings to endure because I know there are toxins in my body that need to be released, but they're trapped. It's as if everything is on an assembly line. Instead of ending up with a finished product, the work is abruptly halted in a stalemate.

Lori has moments when the pain is not so bad. Generally effusive and out-going, when Lori turns inward, her friends question whether she's in pain. "The reason I'm quiet isn't always because I hurt, but because I'm trying to figure out how to patch up my life and dream again. I'm quiet because I have a lot on my mind. It's as if a big part of me has died, and I'm just taking it one day at a time—like someone would mourn the loss of a loved one, except I'm still here."

Lori is wise beyond her years. She speaks to all of us with sexual pain—wisdom from a young woman who has not engaged in sex but has experienced the devastation of the aspects of CPP that disrupt her other relationships and daily life. Her poignant, often poetic, point of view spoke to my heart, as I believe it would to any CPP sufferer.

Lori puts her illness in perspective this way:

> It does trouble me when people complain about mere common colds as if they're dying. However, most of the time, I just figure *everyone* is struggling. They may not be afflicted physically like me, but there are other painful ways to suffer, such as emotionally, spiritually, or mentally.
>
> I'd like to say I never feel sorry for myself, but that would be a lie. Sometimes I just feel so different from everyone else in the world that I begin to envy their health. But then I must remember how many blessings I *do* have in my life, such as my Savior, my family, and my few kindred spirits. Plus, it makes it easier to relate to the lame and blind in the Bible that Christ easily cured with a mere touch. I don't think I have this condition as a punishment, but rather so God's work may be displayed more vibrantly through me.
>
> Sometimes I think that if I pretend the pain isn't there, then maybe I won't feel it, and I can pretend I'm living a *normal* life, whatever that means. Plus, it makes others so much happier to see a cheerful person than a sad person. Nobody asks happy people what's wrong with them. I suppose that is the main reason I pretend to be happy. . . . I'm tired of trying to find the answers to questions that *I* haven't figured out yet.
>
> I hate the looks people give me when they get a glimpse of how horribly my dreams have been shattered. I don't like them feeling sorry for me, and I especially hate feeling like a burden. If I just pretend to be happy all the time, then there isn't room for anyone to ask me, with any real degree of concern, if I'm actually doing well.

Lori admits that she cries easily. One of her doctors told her that she is not suffering from depression because depression is feeling sad for no reason at all, but she has every reason to feel sad. Still, she has sought psychological help, saying,

> The few counselors I have met with have not been very helpful. The first one thought I should allow myself to grieve more about my loss, and when I asked him how long I should grieve, he just scratched his head. The second more qualified one was convinced my disease and issues were just in my head.

The only person who has shed any helpful light on my condition has been my pastor, a wonderful godly man. He just encouraged me to keep seeking the Lord. The way I see it, sometimes what doesn't kill you *does* make you stronger, but sometimes the things that don't kill you just make you more bitter toward life. I'd much rather it be the former.

EARLY PAIN, LATER PROBLEMS

Lori's problems arose in the eighth grade when she began menstruating. She tried to insert a tampon but found it terribly painful. So she used pads instead, but she told no one about the pain because the subject was too embarrassing and she'd found a way around it. However, she soon began having two periods a month and had her first pap smear in ninth grade. The examination itself was extremely painful. The doctor told her she was anatomically small, and no follow-up studies were done regarding the vaginal pain.

Because she was concurrently experiencing constant lower intestinal pain, her mother took Lori to a number of gastroenterologists. All of them diagnosed her with IBS. Early on, she was given an x-ray and said, "They saw stool all the way up to the top of my stomach and just told me to drink prune juice and eat more fiber."

Lori was given cookbooks and, being a perfectionist, she precisely followed directions, keeping her diet regimented. But nothing relieved the pain. "It was disappointing to try so hard, to eliminate the foods I enjoyed, and then feel even worse," she told me.

As time went on, the pain didn't abate, so Lori continued seeing doctors, but they had no new ideas. Finally, when Lori was about 19, she found a doctor who tried to figure out whether her pain emanated from her stomach or was referred to it from her pelvic area.

First, he sent her for a transvaginal ultrasound to determine if she had any cysts. She described the experience. "They couldn't get the probe up me, and it wasn't a big probe at all. They nearly gave me a sedative, but finally got it in. It was excruciatingly painful like my skin was being burned as they stuck the probe in me. I felt like it was stabbing me." Based on her symptoms, the doctor felt confident in a diagnosis of pelvic floor dysfunction but confirmed the diagnosis through a colon study. Lori ingested three capsules with different rings on each and then was x-rayed over the course of a number of days. Based on the results of a specific marker (measuring her gastrointestinal transit time), the doctor's suspicions were confirmed. Lori explained what the doctor told her:

> The muscles in my pelvic area tighten around my intestines and squeeze so hard that it takes a ton of force to actually be able to use the restroom. My pain doctor described my condition as similar to a steel door or a trap door. People like me have

a really, really strong door; it's hard to push stuff out, so that's what most of the medicines are aimed at helping.

According to Dr. Echenberg, "This form of extreme pelvic floor spasm is also the reason that urine won't pass through easily with IC and why anything trying to penetrate the vagina meets resistance. The pelvic floor muscles form a type of sling or hammock. When they're tightly clenched, the urethra, lower bowel, and vagina tighten, and don't easily allow anything in or out."

She said that suffering to the point of debilitation seemed odd to her. "I'm a person who has a really high pain tolerance. I've broken my left foot, my right leg, and my right thumb, and I didn't even cry." She told me she felt relieved when a specialist said that it's typical for people who have high pain tolerance in their outer extremities to have less pain tolerance in their vaginal area.

Among Lori's treatments has been the use of a TENS unit, which she described:

> It's like a stimulator that shoots voltage through my stomach. I had two patches on the front and two on the back. The machine had two settings: a wave and a beating setting. It was supposed to loosen and relax those muscles. It worked for a while, but if I got constipated, it was really painful and I'd have bad cramps and couldn't walk. So they took me off that and, instead, they've been giving me muscle relaxants, like Valium.

Lori was loathe to talk about her problems with anyone other than her mother until she had to wear the TENS unit fanny pack. At that point, she said, "It was just obvious that something was wrong. People would make fun of me and say, 'Oh nice fanny pack.' I'd tell them I had to wear it because I have a neuromuscular disease and my stomach seizes up. In disbelief, they'd say, 'Are you serious?'"

Despite the severity of Lori's own symptoms and the impact it has had on her life, she knows she's lucky to have found help early and understands that her symptoms can progress if they go untreated. She's been told that, eventually, she may become an IC victim. Although she doesn't have that condition yet, she's already prone to frequent bladder infections.

MORE ABOUT HOW LORI'S PARENTS COPE

Lori spoke about her mother, who, before her own diagnosis of IC and pelvic floor dysfunction over two decades ago, was put through a medical meat grinder with a multitude of misdiagnoses. "They treated her like she had STDs; they burned her and did horrible things in an attempt to alleviate the pain. She's been messed with a lot and she's tired of being the guinea pig."

Her dad has stood by her mom's side, saying he'd rather be with her mother, ill though she is, than not have her around at all. Lori said of her mother:

My mom cries sometimes because she realizes how different her life would be if she didn't have this disease. She was very athletic and vibrant. And it breaks my heart that she's not the wife that my dad married. She was carefree and healthy. Now she's weighed down by all these health issues.

Watching her mother's experience has profoundly affected Lori's feelings about her own future and relationships. Lori is not her mother, but her fears, based on a lifetime of seeing and sensing her parent's difficulties as well as her own recent diagnoses, have made her more than cautious.

AFRAID OF THE FUTURE, AFRAID TO LOVE

As a young woman who is not sexually active but hopes to share her life with a man, Lori believes she sees the future when she's probed or "Pap'd" or tries to insert a tampon. She's essentially resigned to not getting married, nor having romance in her life.

"I think relationships are hard in general," she said, "because guys like to fix things, and you can't fix people who are sick. I mean doctors try to, but a boy-friend or a husband feels helpless watching the person he loves suffer." Lori said one of her pain specialists told her that many men end up leaving such relationships because it's so hard to deal not only with the emotional, but the physical issues, in addition to watching someone you love suffer so much.

However, Lori sees her situation as different from her mom's because any man with whom she'd become involved would walk into it knowing she has this condition, whereas her parents had no clue until they'd been married a few years. "My first thought when I was diagnosed was that it wouldn't be fair for some guy to marry me. It wouldn't be fair to limit his life because I'm limited."

Lori has spoken with a few of her closest girlfriends about the vaginal pain she's experienced and her fears about intercourse. "My girlfriends who aren't Christians say, 'That's OK. You can still do this type of sex and that type of sex,' and I just say, 'Yeah, yeah, yeah.'"

But for Lori, thinking about that frustration over a lifetime is difficult to imagine. She's confused but has not completely closed the door to love. Once thinking she'd never get married because no man could handle the situation, she has since recognized that some people, like her dad, see a woman's heart and who she is as a person, not just her physical limitations. Plus, she said, "My parents share the same strong faith."

Of her own faith, Lori said to me, "I never get angry at God. But I do feel a sense of loss sometimes. It's almost like I've lost a part of me, being unable to do certain things."

Lori has never had a serious relationship, saying, "It's ironic because it re-ally has nothing to do with my disease at all. I just have really high standards.

I just haven't met anybody I've been attracted to who has met those ideals." She paused for a moment and added, "Well, I did meet a guy who kind of met those requirements, and then he found out about my pelvic floor dysfunction. We were friends for a while, no more than that. Then the relationship just fizzled out."

Lori confessed she pushed him away because she found herself liking him, explaining, "I didn't want to hurt him because he had just gotten out of a bad relationship." It seemed that her fear of a future permanent relationship, though far off, didn't even allow her to explore the territory in the present.

Unlike many women with CPP who can't function at their job, Lori finds solace in her work as a paralegal, which, she said, requires a great deal of concentrated research but little interaction with others. However, she does find a number of activities daunting, including traveling and socializing. The motion of traveling in a vehicle upsets her stomach, and socializing with friends is challenging because of her extreme food limitations. Therefore, she often isolates herself because it can be overwhelming to deal with the situation and all of her special needs. Lori said her friends want to help, but there is little they can do other than be supportive:

> It isn't a normal illness to have. It isn't as if they can cook for me or bring me some chocolates, because I have trouble digesting nearly everything. Similarly, it isn't as if they could keep my mind off my troubles by taking me out for a drink, because alcohol reacts toxically with my medications and inflames my organs.
>
> I *try* to let people think they're helping me. I give away the chocolates they give me, I pass along the drinks they buy for me, and I come up with all sorts of excuses for why I am the way I am without ever telling them the truth. I sometimes shoo away the people who know what's going on with my body because I don't want to be a burden.
>
> I hate seeing them watch me suffer and not be able to do anything about it, so I just isolate myself when I'm in a great deal of pain.

When she feels better, Lori does push herself to socialize with friends in their environment. She believes it would be unfair to force them to give up their activities due to her disabilities, saying:

> I still go out to the bars and hang out with my close friends. They're respectful of the fact that I can't drink. It's nice of them to still include me.
>
> I've had a lot of guy friends stand up for me when we've gone to bars and other guys offer to buy me drinks. I'll say "no thanks" and they'll say, "What? Are you too good for me?" And then one of my male friends will step in and say, "Hey, she just doesn't drink."

LORI'S MESSAGE: A LOT CAN BE DONE

Lori has advice for young girls with similar problems, saying, "A lot of times, they think, 'this is just something I'm going to have to endure the rest of my life.' But in many cases, a lot can be done." She drew from her own experience with her intestinal issues:

> A diagnosis of IBS was just a blanket term for "you have a stomach problem." Well, I already knew that. Girls shouldn't give up. They should keep trying to figure out exactly what's wrong and find help. One friend of mine jogs and her stomach can't take it. Another always has stomach pains and doesn't know how to deal with it. Neither one has been able to get proper help. They think they can endure it, but there's a big chance it will get worse and they *won't* be able to endure it, so they need to figure it out while they can still be helped.

Chapter Twelve

A TALE OF TWO MEN WHO EXPERIENCE SEXUAL PAIN

While this book is about the relationships of women who suffer, Dr. Echenberg convinced me that it was important to devote a section of *Secret Suffering* to men who experience sexual pain. I was shocked to learn just how similar the experience, pain, and treatment of painful bladder syndrome/interstitial cystitis (PBS/IC) is for men, as well as its devastating effects on their lives and relationships.

Dr. Nel Gerig, urologist, told me about a man who came to her with severe urinary frequency, urgency, pelvic, and testicular pain:

> He talked for 45 minutes, and his wife sat in the corner and cried. Do you know what he said? "If I even think about having sex, it hurts." I asked about musculoskel-etal issues. Is there a back problem? Is there a knee injury? I kept asking and he kept saying no and finally he said, "Oh. There was that fall I had two years ago. I didn't tell you about that. Hiking in the mountains, I fell two feet and landed on a piece of granite. I had a sitting-down injury." Turns out that his body was out of line (pelvic floor dysfunction).

After hearing his story, she sent him to a physical therapist. In two visits with the physical therapist, he showed 85 percent improvement. He had physical therapy in decreasing frequency, until he was able to strengthen the muscles to keep him in line. Today, he plays hockey to keep his structural alignment, though he still goes in for a tune-up. Dr. Gerig is proud to say, "He doesn't have pelvic pain—not anymore. He was a dramatic example of how the musculoskeletal and nerve upregulation components can affect pelvic pain."

Although conventional wisdom seems to indicate that the medical community takes more stock in the veracity of the men they treat, the following stories of Ben and Eric prove that there's clearly a problem across the board when it comes to pelvic pain.

BEN'S STORY

For Ben, the problems started four years ago when he was 25. The onset began when he was at work:

> I got this feeling that I had a urinary tract infection. It started out with painful urination, then burning. As it progressed, it was more pressure than pain, a feeling like I had to urinate even if I had just done so. I went to my family doctor and had a urinalysis, which came back clean. He wasn't sure what to do, so he sent me to a urologist.

And so began Ben's journey to the first of many urologists in search of a diagnosis. Each doctor checked him out thoroughly for any possible cause, including sexually transmitted diseases (STDs). Every test came back normal. Despite no evidence of infection, doctors continually treated him with antibiotics. Ben still wonders why:

> I don't really know what they were treating because there were no bacteria anywhere, but I guess they didn't know what else to do. I took course after course of antibiotics, which didn't help. I went to another urologist for a second opinion.
>
> This doctor, too, was perplexed. The urologist told me that maybe the hole at the tip of my penis was too small and recommended surgery. But luckily that doctor ended up leaving the office and I never followed up with him. I went to yet another doctor who said surgery was unnecessary.

Ben had an IVP test (x-ray of the kidneys) and a cystoscopy (a scope into the bladder and urethra) to see if any cysts or strictures (scars) were present. He also had a bladder ultrasound to check if it was emptying properly. He said, "Some of these tests were extremely unpleasant. I was hoping they would finally diagnose me. But they all just said, 'Nope, everything is normal.' I wanted to yell, 'Well then, what the hell is going on?'"

Because doctors found nothing else, they put Ben back on antibiotics. He'd had previous difficulty with irritable bowel, so he went to a gastroenterologist to see if there was possibly a link between the two conditions. Luckily, the doctor knew enough about PBS/IC to recognize the symptoms and referred him to a pelvic pain expert, who also happened to be a gynecologist! Amazingly, Ben even put aside the obvious embarrassment that must have been present in being asked, as a man, to see a gynecologist.

Symptom-Free at Last

A year and a half after Ben's first symptoms, he finally found a doctor able to treat him. He's been symptom-free for over six months with only one or two flare-ups in the four months prior to that.

In Ben's case, all it took was one doctor educated in spotting the symptoms of IC. Gynecologists, urologists, colorectal surgeons, gastroenterologists, family practitioners—the medical professionals who deal with patients from the waist to the thighs—simply need to take time to become more educated so they can save their patients years of anguish. Ben's gastroenterologist didn't need to treat the problem; he simply had to recognize the symptoms and send his patient to the right specialist.

Ben was lucky. Unlike many who spend a decade or more on the wrong track, he searched for fewer than two years before finding an accurate diagnosis and a doctor who could treat him. Still, he said, "It was long and frustrating—a year and a half of constant pain and no relief."

Ben's physical therapist taught him pelvic strengthening exercises, which helped tremendously. He has continued doing these exercises since being released from physical therapy because they've helped immensely. He's been patient about giving his treatment plan enough time to work, and he told me, "The exercises helped right away, but I would still get flare-ups." Among his medications is Elmiron, which he said, "Didn't fully kick in until I'd been on it for a while," but it has made a significant impact on his pain.

As part of his treatment plan, Ben was given a low-acid diet list. He became very aware of his reaction after eating items on that list, which is how he figured out the foods that bothered him, saying, "I noticed that tomato sauce, like spaghetti and meatballs, definitely affects me, while some of the items on the list don't bother me at all. Like chocolate—that doesn't really bother me. So I just don't eat spaghetti and meatballs as often as I used to, but if I do, I'll take a Prelief with it."

Prelief is an over-the-counter product that is supposed to neutralize the acid in foods and drinks. "Prelief definitely helps with coffee," Ben said. "I have to have my cup every morning and I take Prelief with that. Then the coffee doesn't irritate my stomach at all."

MARRIAGE TESTED

At the time I interviewed Ben, he was going through a divorce. He had met his soon-to-be ex-wife when he was 24, a year before the problems began. They have a two-year-old son.

Ben said, "Before I started having the problem, everything was great as far as my sex life. And then when the pain began, I had no sexual desire whatsoever because I was feeling so uncomfortable down there."

In addition, Ben had difficulty maintaining or even achieving an erection, which he believes was related to his lack of interest and fear of pain. Having an orgasm triggered intense bladder pressure. After sex, he'd strongly feel the urge to urinate, but as he said, "I'd stand there and push and push and I wouldn't be able to go."

Ben felt quite alone in his suffering. He was too embarrassed to talk about it to his close friends because he "felt like an old man," and his wife found it difficult to cope with the situation.

> My wife didn't think this diagnosis of IC was real. At the time, this condition was relatively unknown. She said, "Well, if it's a problem, why don't they just treat it and make you all better?" I told her it's a gradual process and she'd have to be patient.
>
> Before I was diagnosed, she thought I was just making an excuse because I didn't want sex with her. Finally, when I had a diagnosis, at least I could say, "Well, this is the problem."

Ben never brought his wife with him to see the doctor. At home, he would try to force himself to have sex, despite not being in a state of mind to do so. Most often, it didn't work. He tried to show his wife affection and sexually stimulate her so she didn't feel frustrated, but she knew he was forcing himself, which just made her feel worse.

Ben and his wife separated about a year ago when he was starting to feel better. He told me, "Yes, I was feeling better, but I guess other problems had taken over so it didn't really matter at that point." While he doesn't believe that IC was the only factor in their breakup, it was clearly one of the major issues.

In the past year, Ben has been in other relationships. He still has erectile dysfunction and takes Levitra to help out. He explained what his doctor believes is happening for him:

> The urinary pressure isn't there anymore so I have more desire for sex. My doctor thinks I'm just desensitized in that area because of all the previous pain. I had my thyroid and the other standard tests for erectile dysfunction problems. Everything came back normal, so I think his hypothesis makes sense.

Currently, Ben feels the best he has since the problem began. "I feel so much stronger down there. I used to run to the bathroom every hour on the hour. Now I can hold it. I can go to the bathroom three to four times a day without a problem." Where before he had to stop frequently when taking a trip, Ben can travel for a few hours without stopping.

He feels much healthier sexually as well. "My urine stream used to be really weak but now it's a lot stronger. Even when I ejaculate, it's a lot stronger than it used to be. My treatments are helping everything."

As a male, Ben had a heck of a time getting his insurance to pay for his visits to a gynecologist. He told me the doctor's office manager went to great lengths to convince the insurance company that there was no other treatment alternative for him. Happily, he was eventually covered.

What does Ben's story tell us? First, while it's important for patients to question what they're told, finding a doctor to trust—and being willing to test a treatment and continue it when it works—is essential to maintaining a higher quality of life. Second, a male patient shouldn't have to go to the extreme and embarrassing length of seeing a gynecologist to get the help he needs. This further reinforces the desperate need for urologists to become educated in the area of PBS/IC in order to diagnose and treat patients of both genders.

In Dr. Echenberg's Words

PBS/IC appears to occur in women about eight times more than in men, although it may be more prevalent in men than is currently recognized, often because of the lack of educated doctors who, for instance, often misdiagnose it for prostatitis.[1] I, myself, have treated five male patients who were brave enough to seek help from a gynecologist. In most cases, the urologists they saw either had no clue about this diagnosis or were telling their patients they could do nothing to help.

Ben's case appears classic because of three things: (1) his urinary cultures were consistently negative; (2) medications for overactive bladder, the "gotta go, gotta go" disorder of the bladder, had not worked; and (3) he had the typical triad of urinary frequency, urgency, and pelvic/sexual pain that we see in female patients with PBS/IC.

ERIC'S STORY

Eric is 42 years old. When he was 38, he felt a "weird, tingling sensation" on his penis after ejaculation. He tried to ignore it at first, but said, "I started to get inflamed hair follicles on my pelvis, right after ejaculation." The symptoms worsened, as he explained:

> I'd feel a burning sensation on my pelvis and then down my inner thighs. It was especially painful when I sat. My doctor thought I had a yeast infection and he gave me a prescription for cream to rub on it, but that didn't help. Then he sent me to a dermatologist, who said, "I don't know what you have. I don't see anything wrong with your skin."

Every morning, because there was no pressure on his pelvis after sleeping, he felt better. He'd be hopeful that the pain might not erupt, but on his drive to work, it would start up. Eventually, the pain became unbearable, as if he had a severe rope burn on the skin across his pelvis and down his thighs. This was in addition to the inflamed follicles when he ejaculated. Eric said, "I'm an athlete and I have a really high tolerance for pain. But this pain was eating into my skin." In fact, Eric loves extreme sports, such as skiing, mountain biking, kayaking, and rock climbing, but unlike playing through the pain of athletics, his pelvic pain grew too great to withstand.

His family doctor referred him to a urologist, who diagnosed him with prostatitis, an inflammation of the prostate gland. Eric felt relieved. He finally thought he'd get some help. However, the urologist did no testing, just gave him high doses of antibiotics, which, he admits, gave him a break from the pain. After the antibiotics, however, the pain escalated again. He continued seeing the urologist who dismissed his continuing pain as chronic prostatitis, telling him all they could do was experimental surgery. The doctor gave him a lot more medication but never gave him any tests.

Urinary symptoms cropped up. Eric said, "I had to urinate all the time. And it would just trickle out. In addition, my penis wasn't full of blood. It was just like a piece of skin hanging off me. It was kind of weird." So he returned to his family doctor, rage and frustration popping out like those follicles. "I asked him, 'What's wrong with me? I don't know what I have. Do I have some kind of disease, a sexually transmitted disease?' I remember he gave me a shot for gonorrhea, but he never tested me."

At his wit's end, Eric begged the urologist for a referral to someone else who might have a different point of view. According to Eric:

> The doctor literally told me, "We make our money through the surgeries and there are not many doctors who are going to want to see you." I thought, "Screw you, buddy." That was the last time I saw him.

The next family doctor Eric saw thought he'd had an infection that had been treated late. The doctor said it caused nerve damage that triggered pain "when it shouldn't." He was the first doctor to do any significant testing, and he prescribed medication for nerve pain. Eric said, "He tested my urine and blood. He did a prostate exam and actually ruled out prostatitis because it didn't hurt when he applied pressure."

It turned out that Eric had a urinary staph (staphylococcus) infection. Eric said, "When I had an erection it wouldn't be, you know, as robust, and I'd hoped it was caused by the staph infection." He took penicillin, which cured the infection but not the overall problem.

Finding the Right Partner Who Understands

Right around this time, Eric began a romantic relationship. He didn't tell his new girlfriend about his pelvic pain issues, instead, he worked around it, for instance, avoiding sitting down a lot. He was 38 at the time.

Of course, he was concerned about the erectile dysfunction that wasn't going away. His family doctor told him, "It's all in your head." The doctor offered Eric a Viagra prescription. That left Eric feeling demoralized and "weird" because he wasn't even 40 years old, and he'd never had that type of problem.

Finally, through a stroke of luck, his family doctor referred him to a knowledgeable urologist. He was impressed because she did a lot of testing, "and it was kind of funny because I thought it might be uncomfortable with a woman doing a prostate exam on me, but for some reason it just wasn't." She diagnosed Eric with IC and explained it as an inflammation of the bladder wall.

Eric had long since broken up with his girlfriend. Around this time, he met his current wife, Missy, to whom he explained everything. "I told her about the pain, all the symptoms, and the erection problems. There was one time the Viagra didn't work and I couldn't maintain an erection. I was really upset and told her. It was really hard to do. I mean, I'm an emotional person and I was telling her about this really personal thing, so I was worried about her reaction." Missy just held him, told him she loved him, and reassured him that the erection didn't matter.

Eric felt a huge weight lifted from him. He said, "That meant I didn't have to sneak off and take the Viagra. I could say, 'Hey, Missy, are you feeling spunky? Well, OK, I'll go take a little nibble of that pill' and it's not a big deal. That was major."

The urologist put him on medications for his IC, one at a time. Each worked for a while, but nothing truly eliminated the pain. He said:

> I started to get frustrated because, here I was again, taking something that would work for a while, then taking something else that worked for a while. In the meantime, I continued having erection problems. Plus, I'd have some good days and some days I'd experience the pelvic pain down the legs. I was starting to get that pain across my back again, like my lower back would get hot. I'd also get hot and clammy, sweating. That's how Missy knew I was having a bad day.

Eric continued having pain and more tests for his erectile dysfunction. His urologist sent him to a specialist to measure the blood flow in his penis. To do that, he had to sleep with an electronic box attached to his leg with Velcro, with two cloth rings placed around his penis, attached to wires that went back to the box. This contraption would measure his erections at night.

Eric said, "This was demoralizing. You're going to bed with your girlfriend and you have to say, 'Yeah, I'm gonna wear this thing that's measuring my erections.' It sucked. It was really embarrassing. She was super supportive, but still it was humiliating and difficult to do. When I brought the thing back after a week, the doctor said, 'Oh, it didn't measure anything. Can you do this again?'" Eric declined.

How Eric Finally Found Relief

Eric finally found relief from a combination of non-drug therapies. The urologist sent him to a pain specialist who was expert in treating IC patients. He gave Eric an interferential (IF) unit, similar to a TENS unit. (Both machines provide electrical stimulation and are used in physical therapy for a number of conditions, but an IF unit has different current than a TENS unit.) Eric said, "I put on four electrodes, two in my groin and two on my back. The machine was programmed specifically for IC. The doctor's theory was that the pain I experienced was so severe that it tightened up all the tiny little muscles in my pelvic floor and left them in knots. This machine helps stretch them out. Once I started using this machine—BOOM! Instant success."

Eric actually loves wearing the device because of the relief it provides. He's also relieved that it's not another drug. He used to wear it all the time during the day and then cut back when he was at home. Now, he wears it much less. Every now and then, he experiences pain, but it's rare and much less intense than before:

> Most days I don't have pain. And sometimes I get a little glimmer of it but nothing like what I used to have when I'd sit at my desk at work and say, "Boy, I wonder how many more years I can really deal with this? I had a really good quality of life before this mess started, and if this is going to be my life, I don't know if I'm willing to deal with this, it sucks that much."

Eliminating Food Triggers

The other key to recovery for Eric has been eliminating food triggers. He discovered that caffeine, alcohol, and spicy foods bothered him. "I like to have beer every now and then, and I like to drink lattes, and I like spicy food. But I just stopped. I had to." This change in his lifestyle has affected his friendships as well:

> You meet your buddies down at a bar or at dinner and start ordering water instead of beer and they say, "Come on. Drink a beer with me." Slowly I had to explain to people that I get severe pain in my pelvis when I drink alcohol or have caffeine.
>
> At first, I didn't want to explain, but I had to. Especially around alcohol; it always seems people want to drink beer. When I was single, if I was going out on a first date, she'd order a glass of wine and expect I'd want one, too. It's difficult socially.

However, Missy has been Eric's saving grace, even when it came to the food issues. He said, "Missy doesn't drink much. It was ironic that my not drinking was something she found attractive. She was understanding about everything, even my erection problems. Ironically, all my symptoms and the things I needed to do to get healthy were things I thought would hurt a relationship. But in fact, going through all this together has made our relationship stronger."

Eric feels fortunate to have found the doctors he did. About his urologist, he said, "Not only did she have ideas and opinions but she reached out to others she respects for their ideas and opinions. And you know what? It was that combination that got me to where I am. Getting that IF unit was big. I'm also lucky that I had insurance."

However, Eric's negative experiences with the medical community before meeting the urologist who helped him still make him angry. He said:

> To this day, if I have a day when I feel pain, I feel like going back to my first generalist and my first urologist and saying, "I'll see you in court," because it was malpractice for sure. One doctor gave me gonorrhea shots with no test and sent me to a dermatologist who did no tests.
>
> It took my getting in the family doctor's face to get a referral to a urologist. And then that urologist tells me that nobody will want to see me because that's not how doctors make their money.
>
> People grow up thinking doctors take care of you and obviously they're there to make money as well. But come on guys. You docs make great money and you can afford to see people you're not cutting into.

Eric offered advice to men and women who suffer with sexual pain by saying, "You can't treat this type of pain with the mental toughness you'd use in sports. Some of my favorite sports can kill ya', but going through this experience took a lot more out of me than the most treacherous climb ever did."

Instead of trying to weather the turbulent storm of his illness, Eric wished he'd gone for help sooner and been firmer in his demands. His advice is clear: "You need to manage your doctors. You need to push them, challenge them, ask probing questions. You always have to ask, 'Are there tests that can prove that?' Don't just take their word for it."

Chapter Thirteen

OUR RELATIONSHIP WITH THE MEDICAL COMMUNITY: THE DARK SIDE

Nobody would deal with my problem. I've been dismissed by 40 doctors, who basically said, "You've been through all these doctors so why do you keep coming back to me? They've done everything I would do so there's nothing I can do to help you."

—Lois (interviewee)

This has been horribly traumatic. Most doctors didn't know about this problem. They just told me I was getting old and dried up.

—Survey respondent

After all the tests came back negative, the doctors said nothing was wrong. They wouldn't treat the symptoms because they couldn't find the cause. A lot of the doctors felt the need to blame me because they couldn't admit they didn't know what to do.

—Jane (interviewee)

The doctors told me it was all in my head, that I really couldn't be having any pain because I was no longer testing positive for a urinary tract infection and I didn't have endometriosis. I would pray before going to see each new doctor. I'd walk in the office, fingers crossed, thinking, "Please. I don't care if I have cancer at this point. Just tell me it's something so I can learn to deal with it or take steps to make it better. Just tell me it's something."

—Kat (interviewee)

When I first started this project, I thought it would be about love, sex, and intimacy, about relationships with our significant others, period. However, as I interviewed women and their partners, and looked at my own life, it became all too clear that this was a far more complicated topic that included women's relationships with their children, their friends, their employers, and sadly, their health care providers.

The pain women described within the context of sex and intimacy was often dwarfed by their rage at a medical community that has refused to listen to them. Too many doctors have thrown up their hands in frustration, suggesting that these women are so-called problem patients, or worse, hypochondriacs.

In this chapter, we delve into the dark side of patient care. However, there is hope for those who suffer with chronic pelvic pain (CPP) due to the remarkable efforts of a growing number of doctors, researchers, and other health care practitioners who are determined to stand by and heal these patients. The new approach to CPP patient care is explored in the next chapter.

We must look at today's painful reality: the problems many patients experience within our current health care system. For instance, recently, Dr. Echenberg received medical records on a new pain patient in which the previous doctor wrote that she'd inherited this patient from three other physicians who could not figure out a cause for her pain. Doctors pass suffering women off to other doctors to get rid of the problem, often after insisting on invasive testing and, sometimes, despite having no diagnosis, guessing at the cause and giving medications the patient may not need.

In agreement with Dr. Echenberg, Dr. Bruce Kahn, a gynecologist at Scripps Clinic in San Diego, California, acknowledged that he, too, sees many patients after they've been to four, five, or six doctors who put them through diagnostic testing with negative results. As he related, "Too often, the patient is told there is nothing physically wrong and that it must all be in your head, which is the worst thing doctors can do. That's the old school way of thinking: it's either in the mind or in the body. But the mind and the body are intricately bound together."

LAUREN'S RUNAROUND

Lauren was diagnosed with vulvar vestibulitis and has a vivid memory of the first time she experienced the pain. She said, "We were in Florida, coming from a colder climate, and I changed into shorts. Suddenly, my clothes felt tight and I got kind of a rubbing sensation in the vulvar area. I didn't think much about it except to keep pulling the clothes away from my genitals."

Over the next six months, Lauren tried every over-the-counter preparation she could find to calm the inflamed feeling. Finally, she went to her family doctor, who did an in-office urine test and said, "Yeah, maybe there's a little bit of a bladder infection." Lauren took a course of antibiotics, but it didn't help. She continued to suffer throughout the summer, telling herself, "Well, it's the heat. It's the moisture."

A month later, she went back to the doctor who then *guessed*, without any further testing, that Lauren might have a yeast infection and put her on anti-fungal medication. The medicine caused a severe flare-up of her symptoms, so she discontinued it. She returned to the doctor every month for another year. At one point, she said, "The gynecologist told me I had unresolved anger. She made me feel awful."

Yes, I imagine by that point, Lauren, as all of us who have experienced such inept care and misdiagnoses, might have a little bit of unresolved anger, anger that could easily erupt at the next poor sap with a medical license who knowingly or unknowingly leads her down the wrong path. I think most of us don't express our feelings to these doctors. Most of us just walk out of the office and kick the proverbial dog. After all, the doctors are the professionals and I, for one, am intimidated by that very expensive degree that must mean the people telling me I'm crazy, or that it's a psychological issue, know what they're talking about.

Yet another year passed during which doctors told Lauren over and over they couldn't see anything wrong. However, they continued to give her antibiotics "just in case," after doing every possible test (twice) to rule out venereal disease, bacterial infection, and so on. The results always came back negative.

Lauren expressed the frustration so many of us have experienced in our journey to get help, "You can't see a headache, you can't see neuropathy, you can't see a whole lot of other things that people have, like backaches. You can't see them, but they're real. They're very real."

The last gynecologist she saw before becoming a patient of Dr. Echenberg prescribed a suppository for yeast. She said, "When I used it, it felt like fireworks exploded inside me. When I went back, she looked at me, folded her arms, and said, 'I really don't know what to tell you, so I'm going to send you to another doctor.'"

And that's when she met Dr Echenberg. She now feels significantly better. For Lauren, it was a miracle to finally find a doctor who believed her, provided a diagnosis, and could treat her CPP.

HYSTERIA: AN INSULT TO WOMEN

Prior to a talk that Dr. Echenberg gave on CPP, one of the gynecologists present asked, "In your practice, don't you predominantly see hysterical drug-seekers?" This is an unfortunate misconception and a sad commentary on the views of some doctors regarding patients who complain of pain that may not be seen on examination.

Dr. Kahn trains doctors on how to effectively work with CPP patients. He has also found that when a new patient comes in complaining about chronic sexual or pelvic pain, doctors may become concerned that the patient is pretending to have pain just to convince the doctor to prescribe drugs. He dis-abuses them of that notion by teaching them that chronic pain, which often cannot be seen, should not be judged through the lens of the acute model of pain (such as a patient coming in with a broken arm).

According to Dr. Karen J. Berkley, neuroscientist and pelvic pain researcher, when patients insist they are in pain, it's true, even if it's not apparent to an outside observer and even if the person appears to be functioning just fine. She said, "If a person says on a scale of 0 to 10 that their pain is a 10, it's a 10. The question is, how and why is she getting to that 10?" In rare circumstances, it might be an attempt to obtain pain medications such as opioids, but Dr. Berk-ley said the patient might not be lying about the severity of her pain, even in that case, because the nervous system is determining priorities, and so, to the patient, the pain feels like a 10.

This idea of the hysterical patient reminded me of the attitude toward women in the Victorian Era. At that time, if a female patient came to the doctor with symptoms such as feeling faint or nervous, with insomnia, fluid retention, muscle spasms, shortness of breath, irritability, loss of appetite for food or sex, and a tendency to cause trouble, they were diagnosed with so-called female hysteria.[1]

The so-called cure for these patients was often manual stimulation by the doctors to induce what we now know as orgasm. In the early twentieth cen-tury, this diagnosis was, thankfully, no longer popular. The disgraceful treat-ment some women suffer at the hands of the medical community today is simply the twenty-first-century equivalent of this outrageous invalidation of female pain.

Earlier, I wrote about the 77-year-old woman who called me, desperate for help to relieve her vaginal burning, telling me she wanted to die because it hurt so badly. She told me her son found our Web site. *Her son!* Imagine how severe the pain must have been to confide such a personal problem to her own son. She called me because she's seen so many doctors who insisted there was nothing wrong with her and didn't know where to turn. I felt help-less. All I could do was refer her to Web sites that had lists of doctors in her state. It was nothing really, but by the end of our conversation, she told me she felt better just knowing she wasn't alone and that she had been able to speak with someone who had the same problem, someone who didn't think she was imagining her pain.

HEALTH CARE PROFESSIONALS ARE PEOPLE, TOO

To be fair, some of the experts with whom I spoke provided a different point of view regarding dedicated practitioners who inadvertently fail their patients. In our struggle for relief, sometimes it's hard to see the other side, but doctors, after all, are people too, with egos and hearts and a limit to frustration. That's often forgotten when, as a patient, you feel desperate for help, and especially when the physician's frustration is misdirected at you.

Dr. Lyndsay Elliott, clinical psychologist, admitted that caring for CPP patients generally challenges physicians, saying, "It's a very defeating process, not only for the patient but for the physician as well. It can take a long, long time for these patients to get better, and it's often easier just to go on to the next patient with whom the doctor can feel successful."

The late Dr. C. Paul Perry, gynecologist and medical director for the C. Paul Perry Pelvic Pain Center in Birmingham, Alabama, explained that most doctors who go into OB/GYN do so for the gratification they get from deliveries and from operating on patients with acute conditions where there can be complete recovery. Addressing the reticence of doctors to treat CPP patients, he surmised, "The number one reason is that doctors just don't have any magic bullets. They don't know what to do with these patients, so they're very uncomfortable. In the surveys I'm familiar with, only 17 percent of gynecologists said they enjoyed taking care of chronic pelvic pain patients."

In alignment with Dr. Perry, Dr. Daniel Brookoff, oncologist and director of the Center for Medical Pain Management at Presbyterian-St. Luke's Medical Center in Denver, Colorado, said, "Some doctors either don't feel there's a treatment or they're afraid of the treatments that are out there. And that's how doctors deal with a disease they can't treat: They run away."

UNDERSTANDING IS THE KEY TO EFFECTIVE TREATMENT OF CPP

Dr. Echenberg feels that most physicians do not yet understand that the pain itself is the diagnosis. The typical reaction of a physician who can't find the cause of a specific set of symptoms is frustration and sometimes anger, which might be perceived by the patient as being directed toward her. Part of the problem is that doctors have been taught to focus primarily on acute pain, and they have not been properly educated in the treatment of chronic pain. In addition, treating chronic pain is a time-consuming challenge.

Chronic pelvic pain is a miserable, treacherous, veiled enemy to overcome. The key to treating CPP is to realize that the pain is itself the diagnosis and that doctors have to find those nerve, muscle, and organ triggers, which may not seem obvious to the uneducated doctor. In addition, doctors are not traditionally trained to look at the sum of the parts. Instead, they're taught how to treat acute conditions and may be inappropriately educated or uninterested in figuring out complex, chronic disorders where multiple symptoms, systems, and organs might be connected. Therefore, the urologist can get rid of your kidney stones and the gynecologist can perform a vestibulectomy or treat endometriosis (medically or surgically), but if the pain persists, a doctor who doesn't understand CPP won't realize that a complex web of nerves, muscles, ligaments, and organs must all be addressed. Therefore, the patient is most often left abandoned.

This is the problem with the à la carte method of sexual pain management today. Each symptom/condition treated individually will never resolve the whole. All treated at the same time can result in tremendous overall improvement.

In Dr. Echenberg's Words

Before coming to see me, the average patient has already endured multiple surgical and invasive diagnostic procedures, such as ultrasounds, MRIs, CT scans, colonoscopies, cystoscopies, laparoscopies, hysterectomies (even under the age of 25), lasering or cauterizing endometriosis implants, surgical removal of structures including gall bladder, appendix, ovarian cysts, adhesions, and so forth that sometimes may leave them worse off than ever. There is a time and place for all of these valuable procedures, and women may often benefit greatly from them. However, the health care system doesn't blink at spending hundreds or thousands of dollars on each of these procedures, but it may not cover adjunct therapies that could help CPP patients, such as pelvic floor physical therapy, acupuncture, myofascial trigger point therapies, and so forth. Therefore, patients who desperately need some of these treatments cannot afford them.

OBSTACLES TO CARE

We need to fundamentally change the mindset of health insurance companies so they understand that preventive medicine is far less expensive in the long run. This era of managed health care engenders decreasing reimbursements from insurance carriers, defensive medicine due to mounting medical-legal suits, and little incentive for care providers to spend quality time listening to women's experiences of their own bodies. Is it surprising that the system actually dissuades practitioners from dealing effectively with the complexities of CPP patients?

Even the doctors who have the passion and willingness to work with these patients, or researchers who engage in long-term research to find a cure or reduce the complex symptoms that cause sexual pain, express their own frustration. They have to deal with a medical system that doesn't encourage persistence to take these issues seriously, doesn't promote education for better diagnoses and treatments, and discourages doctors from spending adequate time with suffering patients.

JANE SUFFERED HUMILIATION BEFORE SHE TRIUMPHED

Jane's story is the perfect example of misdirected frustration, misdiagnosis, and disrespectful treatment at the hands of doctors. Her primary condition is interstitial cystitis (IC). Jane's symptoms started in the early 1980s with urinary frequency and urgency. By 1993, she said, "Pain would shoot from my lower back down into the labia, and I had this heavy feeling, like everything was going to fall out the bottom."

For the next nine years, Jane found herself on a diagnosis-seeking crusade. Along the way, she had multiple CT scans, MRIs, x-rays, and four laparoscopies. When they all came back negative, doctors told her nothing was wrong. She felt like killing herself. Jane described one especially humiliating experience when she was admitted to the hospital with agonizing pain:

> At one point, I called for the night nurse. The doctor had given an order for a morphine drip every four hours. When she came in, she read me the riot act about how I was getting too much medication and said, "I don't know if anyone has told you, but all your tests are negative."
>
> They sent in a psychiatrist accompanied by a group of interns. He asked me how often I smoked marijuana in college. I hadn't. He continued asking a number of very unpleasant, personal, and embarrassing questions.
>
> They walked out, and right in front of my door, I heard the psychiatrist say to them, "If anybody under 50 tells you they've never smoked marijuana, you can assume they're lying and therefore, you can assume they're inclined to lie about their drug use. I want you to call her pharmacy and find out what she's been taking."

Today, the pain is bearable for Jane at night if she wakes up every two to three hours to go to the bathroom. But if she sleeps for more than six hours, she can't move. "I have to grab the heating pad and put it on for 15 minutes before I can get up and go to the bathroom because it feels like I'm bursting. But when I finally get to the bathroom, it's just drip, drip, drip. My bladder is in spasm."

Jane understands that managing her condition, not curing it, is the goal. She believes Dr. Echenberg saved her life with proper diagnosis and appropriate treatment. Now she wishes she could blast all those other doctors:

> I'm angry that it took nine years to get a diagnosis. I saw *so many* doctors in that time. And I told them I had pelvic pain. Nobody ever asked me about urinary symptoms, and that includes urologists.
>
> Doctors do need to ask people complaining of pelvic pain whether they have their appendix. But immediately after that, they should ask how many times you get up at night to pee. I had frequency for so long it never occurred to me to associate it with the pain. I just accepted I had a little bladder and that's the way it was.

Because she understands that doctors don't have all the answers ("Well, we haven't cured cancer and AIDS"), her anger is not so much about lack of knowledge as lack of humane and fair treatment. She explained:

> Doctors take women less seriously than they take men. My husband agrees with me. Every time I've taken him with me to a doctor or a hospital, I've been taken care of more quickly and more seriously, and I've gotten better care. It's infuriating.

> Often when my husband is in the examination room with me, the doctor will talk to *him* about my symptoms, as if I'm two years old and incapable of answering. I feel like saying, "Hello! Do you want him to take off his pants so you can address your questions directly to his penis?"

The worst blow to Jane was hearing from doctors how healthy she looked, as she recalled, "Well, yeah. I've always had pink cheeks and bright blue eyes . . . and now I'm being punished for it. I just don't know how to look less healthy."

She's right. One of the ironic misfortunes of CPP is that many woman do look the picture of health, which sometimes makes it difficult for doctors, significant others, friends, family, and coworkers to believe their suffering is real.

THE BLADDER AS A BIG AND COMMON TRIGGER

When Dr. C. Lowell Parsons, professor of surgery at the University of California at San Diego, California, first began practicing urology, female patients would present with what were supposed to be recurrent bladder infections. As previously noted, his earlier research showed the bladder was resistant to infection,[2] and he found that these patients weren't suffering from infections at all but from IC. He said, "Having infections is a myth propagated by the big pharmaceutical companies making $3.5 billion selling antibiotics. IC is not rare. It's very common, and most of my patients had been misdiagnosed by gynecologists." How many have labeled it "honeymoon cystitis," or just associated with sex, when cultures come back negative?

Dr. Parsons believes that proper diagnosis is often missed because doctors don't see the association between the symptoms:

> If you're a 20-year-old woman having pain with sex or pelvic pain the week before your period, then which specialist would you see? If you see a gynecologist, you'll get a gynecologic diagnosis because that's their paradigm. The fact that you're going to the bathroom 14 times a day gets completely missed unless they give you the Pelvic Pain and Urgency/Frequency Patient Symptom Scale (PUF). [See Appendix B.]
>
> If they start to focus in on the bladder as the generator of the symptoms, they'll find out that many of their patients have urinary frequency and urgency with their pain. At that point, the gynecologist will have learned that patients have urinary frequency and they've also been diagnosed with vulvodynia, for instance, so they see an association.

But Dr. Parsons goes one step further. He insists, "They're not associated, *they're the same problem.*"[3] Dr. Echenberg said, "When I first started to investigate all of the reasons for CPP by reading the new texts and searching the medical literature, as well as going to conferences on pelvic pain, it became more and more clear to me that painful bladder syndrome (PBS), otherwise known as interstitial cystitis (IC), and irritable bowel syndrome together are major triggers for CPP in at least 60 to 70 percent of patients. In fact only 20 percent of CPP can be attributed to gynecologic pathologies alone. This came as a shock and revelation to me as a practicing gynecologist for over 30 years."[4]

LOIS'S SURGERY FROM HELL

Lois is one such patient who found the compassion of a caring doctor made all the difference, but her path to finding him was strewn with the rocks and boulders of bad care over which many of us have stumbled on our way. In an earlier chapter, you read about Lois's sudden pain on the boardwalk where she stumbled and thought her underwear was too tight. Her doctor had prescribed pain pills to treat tendonitis. That was the moment she began her descent into the hell of sexual and pelvic pain.

Her daily activities were accompanied by a constant burning in her genital area. After the pain pills didn't work, she hit an immediate brick wall in her search for help, leaving her emotionally bloodied and bruised.

> I called the family doctor back a couple of weeks. The nurse told me that the doctor would return my call. I waited a week to call again. The nurse said she'd put a note on his desk.
>
> Another week passed before I called to let the nurse know that I still had heard nothing. I was very polite.
>
> About a half hour later, my phone rang and I heard this doctor raving at me, saying such things as "How dare you yell at my nurse about this?" He ended the conversation by telling me, "I have better things to do than deal with your pain. People who are really sick need my time." And that was the end of him.

She saw a cadre of doctors, including department heads of the most renowned universities and medical centers, including gynecologists, an oncologist, and a urogynecologist. No one had any answers for her.

In 1997, Lois and her husband, Gus, found one of the few doctors who would perform a pudendal nerve release surgery. He lived halfway across the country, but based on the reassuring advice of her local gynecologist, Lois and Gus believed surgery would put an end to her pain problem. Unfortunately, this wasn't the case:

> The surgery lasted three hours. I had trouble coming out of the anesthesia so it ended up being a six or seven hour ordeal for me before I even came to. The next day, when I sat up, the pain was still there.

Here's how she described her conversation with the doctor the morning after the surgery:

He said everything had indicated the pudendal nerve was part of my problem, but the success rate for this procedure was not guaranteed. It was something they were testing. I think he said around 50 percent of women had positive results. I was in the other 50 percent. I headed back to Pennsylvania in a lot of discomfort because of the operation *plus* my original pain.

It would have been nice if the referring doctor had told her this *before* the procedure so their hopes would have been tempered with a strong dose of skepticism to keep their enthusiasm in check.

Gus found the situation infuriating. They expected a certain amount of post-operation pain and recovery, but the pain never got better. To make matters worse, when she returned to her home doctor, he sent her spiraling further down the black hole of despair by telling her, "Well, if he can't help you, I can't help you."

Gus added, "It was so aggravating. Some of the doctors said there was a lot of scar tissue from a previous course of steroid injections and that was probably the cause of her pain. We bought that for a while. Then, some other doctors disagreed with that theory."

She'd been dismissed by 40 doctors: Dr. Echenberg was number 41. Gus said, "At least he understands, and he is tender and respectful. That's the problem we were having. Other doctors have just gone in there and poked and rammed. Not peaceful at all."

Lois said, "Dr. Echenberg was willing to listen and didn't slough me off by saying, 'Well if this doesn't work then I don't know what to do.' He's constantly trying different things to see what will alleviate or lessen my pain. He makes every patient feel important."

In Dr. Echenberg's Words

Not long ago, Lois saw one of the top surgeons currently performing pudendal nerve release surgery. He immediately recognized that her scar was indicative of the approach that some of the earliest doctors in the United States had used, and he explained that this surgery was no longer being done because they eventually found it ineffective. A less invasive procedure showing results that are more positive has been developed. Testing did reveal that her pudendal nerve might be released from this new surgery, but to date, she has not made the decision to chance it again.

We are still treating her with medications and periodic pudendal blocks. Lois has remained fairly stable and is able to function with her routine activities. It is also important to note that most of our patients are maintained or significantly improved with conservative nonsurgical approaches.

SUSPENDING DISBELIEF

Sandy DiDona, Dr. Echenberg's nurse, agreed that it is very difficult for doctors to believe what they cannot see, especially when the acute model of pain management belies this. She said:

> Doctors are challenged to suspend disbelief when hearing their patients' complaints, since so many CPP patients don't look like they are in pain. But they must do so. They have to understand that patients are so used to having the condition, they've learned to mask it. It's our hope that all physicians will learn to recognize the symptoms of pelvic pain despite their patients' appearance. They can do this by just asking a few questions to see if their patient fits the mold.

Tiffany and Samantha are both in their early 20s and are both patients of Dr. Echenberg. They, too, have experienced the problem with looking too healthy. Tiffany said, "Usually I'd get dressed up when I went to the doctor's office, so the doctor wouldn't think I looked sick. But what doctors don't understand is that you may look great, but you feel terrible. They don't understand that it takes so much energy just to function. This disease takes so much out of you."

Samantha said, "Tiffany and I both got to the point where no doctor listened to us, so we thought, OK, we'll wear sweatpants and a sweatshirt and no makeup. Maybe if we look the part, if we look sick, then they'll take us seriously. That's how profoundly discouraging it was to have no one listening to either of us. And our plan didn't even work."

It's infuriating for patients who walk into the doctor's office filled with hope to leave still in pain, and now dejected, angry, and even more confused, as if, somehow, it's their fault that the pain doesn't show.

PATIENTS ARE NOT JUST BODY PARTS

Perhaps the most frustrating question about CPP is: Why doesn't the medical community get it so we can get the help we need? Why don't medical practitioners understand that there's an epidemic of pain destroying the lives of women, shredding the fabric of intimacy for millions of couples, which surely contributes to the high divorce rate in this country? Why don't they understand the urgency of working harder to find an answer?

The experience of Dr. Berkley offers some insight. It has been a lengthy scientific process by researchers such as Dr. Berkley to sort out the pieces of the puzzle as to how injurious or potentially injurious stimulus information is received and processed by the central nervous system. She believes that these inconsistencies in the clinical world of medicine in understanding the interrelationships she has uncovered are due in large part to our health care system segmenting the different organs of our bodies as separate entities. Dr. Berkley said:

> We can forget that what makes an entire individual work as a functioning whole is our nervous system. It's always adjusting things. If we lean over, we don't fall down because of all these automatic adjustments of our nervous system (such as which muscles are contracting and which muscles are relaxing). We don't notice and it's not conscious. The nervous system, in essence, coordinates all that we take in and all that we do. If we didn't have that kind of controlling system, we'd just be a bunch of different body parts that would not work in harmony.

Dr. Berkley believes that more and more members of the medical community are increasingly thinking of patients holistically, instead of just a conglomeration of body parts. Dr. Echenberg agrees, and his hope is that this new scientific understanding of the nature of pain will spread quickly to specialists and primary care physicians alike, who are regularly approached by patients with chronic pelvic pain and sexual pain disorders.

Her enthusiasm about the results of her team's research was apparent in our interview. "We're at a point right now where we're finding things out left and right. It's coming so fast. We're learning information that we're really excited about. The research is giving us insights into conditions like pelvic floor dysfunction and vulvodynia." Dr. Berkley's groundbreaking work is paving the way for better pelvic and sexual pain treatment, and maybe even a cure one day.

LIVING WITH CPP: SUSAN'S JOURNAL

It was music to my ears to hear that the wave of the future of medicine, at least regarding CPP, was to look at patients holistically. I was all for whatever it would take for doctors to finally see me as a complete entity instead of parts, like a carburetor or transmission. My own experience validated that bizarre separation of body, mind, and spirit by the medical community. Case in point:

1. The internist sent me to the gastroenterologist to check out my stomach, who found essentially nothing wrong.
2. Innumerable gynecologists who had me on rounds and rounds of antibiotics, until I went to the immunologist who did extensive testing and explained that these weren't infections, and I was creating far more problems by taking the antibiotics than not. (The immunologist was right. Now, I insist on cultures first and haven't had to take an antibiotic for a vaginal infection in years.)
3. The psychiatrist dealt with my brain but said no pill could change my personality (whatever *that* meant), and I would have to work out my other issues with a therapist.
4. The therapist helped me gain some insights but didn't help my pain at all (or change my intense personality one bit, to the disappointment of my husband).

5. The sex therapist insisted it was all psychological and suggested a set of expensive dildos to relax my muscles (which I couldn't afford at the time). She never asked any of the questions that would have alerted her to what was contributing to the pain (which was physical).

6. The vulvodynia specialist at a prestigious hospital did a quick exam and (incorrectly) determined that I didn't have vulvodynia.

7. At least the next gynecologist did a Q-tip test. When I jumped through the roof at "10 P.M.," she said, "You have vestibulitis." This diagnosis was accurate, but it was unfortunately only one of many issues contributing to my sexual pain.

8. I asked one or two of the specialists I'd seen regarding my many assorted ailments whether all my symptoms could possibly be related. To a person, their eyes glazed over and they each said (in their own special way) that they only specialize in whatever part of me had been put on the table for checking.

9. And last, but not least, there was the well-known, highly respected urologist who was brusk and rather nasty. He wouldn't even look at the records I brought him from Dr. Echenberg about my case, and he snickered at the idea of bladder instillations.

   He did do one test to see how I was voiding, which came out fine, so to speak. Despite all that I told him, he insisted I needed two very expensive and invasive procedures for him to ensure I had IC. Sorry to say, I could practically see the dollar signs in his eyes.

   And there was no doubt in my mind, as I sat there on the verge of tears, that if they came back negative, he would be just another doctor who would shrug and say, "Sorry, there's nothing wrong with you." Maybe those procedures would have been good diagnostic tools. Maybe not. But I wasn't going to let such a callous doctor touch me.

   During my exam, to make matters worse, he brought in two other young doctors who witnessed this treatment, and he talked to them about me as if I wasn't there. So here is the rub. Doctor "Expert" passes on his attitude to "New" doctor so that, just as Pavlov's dogs, they learn that this is an acceptable way to treat patients. Well, Dr. Nasty, it isn't.

Needless to say, I feel victorious that the idea of a whole body–whole person approach and a philosophy of kindness toward the patient's body, mind, and spirit, so long sneered at by the mainstream medical community, turns out to be the path to healing CPP after all.

The good news is that, despite all the brick walls, an ever-growing (albeit still too small) community of exceptional gynecologists, physician researchers, physical therapists, psychiatrists, urologists, alternative therapists, and other representatives from the medical research community have devoted themselves to solving the puzzle of CPP. A common thread among these professionals is their determination to continually and thoroughly educate themselves about treating chronic pelvic pain. The International Pelvic Pain Society is a perfect example of such a group of dedicated and multidisciplinary professionals.

HOW ONE WOMAN MADE A DIFFERENCE

Dr. Brookoff was trained as an oncologist, but he is now one of the most respected pain management specialists and a hero in the IC world. The course of Dr. Brookoff's career was altered by the words of one woman.

In 1978, Dr. Brookoff was a medical student at the University of Pennsylvania. During the course of a few urology lectures, one small segment was devoted to IC. He said, "The professor basically told us, 'These women are crazy. They're old ladies. Honestly, eventually you have to take out their bladders. But it's all in their heads. If you ever see them, they'll ask you for pain medicine. Turn around and run.'"

Dr. Brookoff remembered that one of the few women in the class raised her hand and asked, "If it's all in their heads, why are you taking out their bladders?" The professor politely told her to shut up and ended the lecture. This was the sum total of IC training Dr. Brookoff received in medical school.

A number of years later, he became an oncologist and didn't think much about IC until he met Denise and her sister Janet:

> A patient came to me in terrible pain from breast cancer; she had a mass growing out through her chest. The idea of having cancer is terrible and chemotherapy is frightening, so many take a third pathway: they try to deny it away. Both Denise and her husband were in serious denial. Even though she hadn't told anybody, her family members knew something was drastically wrong. I put her in the hospital, where she was put on a pain pump. After that, she brightened up and welcomed her family, who came to support her.

Her sister Janet took Dr. Brookoff aside. She saw how much better Denise was feeling and thought it was the chemotherapy. However, she hadn't started chemotherapy yet, and Dr. Brookoff told her, "Relieving Denise's pain brought her back to herself."

Then Janet said, "Well, I have a painful disease. Can you treat me? I have a disease called interstitial cystitis." Dr. Brookoff remembered the lecture all those years ago. He remembered the professor saying, "Don't touch those people!" So he told her:

> "Janet, I'm an oncologist. I don't really know much about IC." We had some famous urologists where I practiced. I named them and she said, "I've seen all of them."
> I said, "To be honest, I just don't feel comfortable. I don't know much about the disease. I really only treat cancer." And she looked me dead in the eye and said, "Well then, in that case, I wish I had cancer."

Dr. Brookoff said there are two kinds of religious moments in life. One where you know God is standing next to you and one where you think He isn't. He said:

That moment was one of the latter. That was a moment where it shook me to my core that someone told me she thought having cancer was a step up from her own illness.

I said, "Let me look into this and give me a couple days to think about it. Neither of us is going anywhere." I read up on IC. I spoke to the urology doctors and they were really kind of dismissive about it. I thought seriously about what to do. So I began taking care of her and she did really well. Then I started seeing her friends.

And that is the story of how one woman who was at the end of her rope found the courage to demand help; she changed the life of not only one doctor, but hundreds of patients.

Chapter Fourteen

INTO THE LIGHT: THE NEW PARADIGM OF CHRONIC SEXUAL AND PELVIC PAIN TREATMENT

I think what's made our clinic successful is that the doctors in our community and in surrounding cities and states don't feel that we're trying to steal their sheep. We don't want their sheep. We want to do what we can to help doctors control their patients' pain and then send them back for routine care.

—The late Dr. C. Paul Perry

After three months of treatments, my pain was almost non-existent. I can sit and not have to shift my weight every five minutes. And intercourse has become more regular and enjoyable again! So after a long two and a half years of not knowing, and second guessing my pain and body—I am fixed, thanks to Dr. Echenberg.

—Victoria (interviewee)

I wish I would have learned about Dr. Echenberg's treatment plan 10 years ago, so I wouldn't have had to suffer as long as I did. If it wasn't for his treatment plan and physical therapy, I don't know where I would be today. I keep thinking, "Wow, five months of treatment just took away a lifetime of pain!"

—Kim (interviewee)

According to Dr. Echenberg, the key to successfully treating chronic pelvic pain (CPP) is to realize that the pain is itself the diagnosis and to find and treat the triggers. The truth is, the pelvis is the busiest area of the body, with all kinds of organs, muscles, ligaments, and nerves. Problems in one or more of these areas can mix and match in any configuration to trigger sexual and pelvic pain disorders. It's still a puzzle, but the difference is that now there's an overall philosophy, proven research, and medical treatments that greatly increase the odds that a properly handled patient will experience significant improvement in all areas of her life, including her most intimate.

It's beyond the purview of *Secret Suffering* to offer specific treatment approaches, although some of the more common have been noted throughout the stories of interviewees and the comments of experts. However, we feel that treatment options would be best discussed with your doctor. Therefore, this chapter provides an overview of the new system that will enable patients to get the best possible treatment, rather than specific medications and procedures.

The new model of CPP treatment is based on a nonsurgical approach to diagnosis and management. Dr. Echenberg sends women for surgery only as a last resort and when all other options have been exhausted, because too many of his patients have been referred to him after experiencing unsuccessful surgery or unnecessary invasive procedures. Dr. Bruce Kahn, a gynecologist at Scripps Clinic in San Diego, California, agreed, saying, "I perform a lot of gynecologic surgery. However, very few of my patients with chronic pelvic pain need surgery."

Dr. Echenberg said:

> This new modality (nonsurgical approach) is based on findings that a significant percentage of diagnostic laparoscopies and other invasive and costly diagnostic studies traditionally yielded either negative or minimally positive findings. Therefore, most of our patients are maintained or significantly improved with conservative nonsurgical approaches.

Dr. Echenberg's vision is to initially encourage urologists, gastroenterologists, gynecologists, and other doctors who are most likely to have been approached by CPP patients to become trained in this specialty when they no longer do surgery or are approaching retirement. These are the doctors who have the background and time to build on their decades of experience.

There is one caveat: Doctors who embark on this journey must have the temperament to deal with angry, frustrated, and irritable patients on a daily basis. According to Dr. Echenberg, "The payoff is that there have never been more gratifying moments professionally than being able to significantly improve the quality of these people's lives. Because of this, the morale of the doctor, patients, families, and staff remain extremely positive and high, in spite of the degree of difficulty in working on these complex medical problems."

Doctors are desperately needed in this specialty. Right now, there are too few doctors to take care of all the CPP patients who need help. The practices of all of the experts with whom I spoke are overflowing with patients. The C. Paul Perry Pelvic Pain Center in Birmingham, Alabama, is kept full strictly by referrals from other doctors.

According to Dr. John F. Steege, gynecologist and professor and chief of the Advanced Laparoscopy and Pelvic Pain division, Department of Obstetrics and Gynecology at the University of North Carolina at Chapel Hill, "One thing we try not to do is treat people who travel great distances because it just doesn't satisfy anybody."

I told him about my own frustrated experiences finding help locally and that of other women with whom I've spoken, and I asked him, "If there's no help, what are we going to do?" Dr. Steege said, "That's the problem. There are some medical wastelands in the country. We do get people from such places every once in a while, but trying to find somebody for them to go back to. . . . It's just really hard."

EDUCATING DOCTORS

Without understanding how to recognize the signs of chronic pelvic pain, even the most diligent and compassionate doctor will prove of little help to the patient. A doctor educated in the current treatment of pelvic pain will know the right questions to ask to properly diagnose the patient. Furthermore, a doctor interested and educated in pelvic pain is less likely to give up on a patient because he would have an arsenal of tools to help the patient find relief.

I asked Dr. Perry what needs to happen to align the number of doctors who can diagnose and treat CPP with the growing population of women who suffer with it. Dr. Perry said that the International Pelvic Pain Society (IPPS) was established to disseminate such education to doctors of all specialties and has been a great benefit to cross-pollinate with other medical disciplines because CPP is not just a gynecological problem. He continued:

> There are very few pain residency programs that train on chronic pelvic pain, even though at least 20 percent of the patients these doctors see every day are chronic pelvic pain patients.
>
> Our main tool is trying to get people to come to meetings to learn about chronic pelvic pain, the causes, the physiology of it, the neurophysiology of it, the psychology of it, and the available treatments.

Dr. Perry's clinic is associated with a network of off-site specialists. If it's determined that the patient needs a pain psychologist, gastroenterologist, urologist, and so forth, such providers who understand the nature of CPP are just a phone call away. But, he cautioned, "You have to know a little bit about all those specialties yourself to know how to refer." This is why education is key for the gynecologist or other specialist working with CPP patients.

For instance, when urinary symptoms, such as frequency, first present themselves, rather than simply prescribing antibiotics, doctors can routinely do cultures first. If negative, they can learn the right questions to ask to guide them to the appropriate treatment or specialist to deal with the problem at the onset.

KNOWING WHEN AND WHERE TO REFER PATIENTS

While a single doctor (usually the gynecologist) must be the quarterback, managing the patient's care, it is rare that one doctor alone can provide the entire range of treatment for the complexities involved with CPP. Using a multidisciplinary approach (incorporating the skills of other doctors or specialists within a treatment plan) encourages a more cooperative relationship between medical professionals, which is a vital aspect to effective management of CPP. This way of managing patients is gaining momentum and proving successful in treating women with chronic pelvic and sexual pain on a physical and emotional level and restoring their quality of life and relationships.

Lisa Iacovelli is a physical therapist who gets many referrals from doctors who have difficulty managing pelvic pain patients, and she welcomes them. The good news is that now she has developed a network of practitioners, such as urologists and gynecologists, who get together regularly to learn about CPP from each other. Instead of sending patients to her out of frustration, she now works *with* the doctor to treat the patient. Lisa is adamant about the importance of such an approach:

> This sharing of expertise really helps with chronic pain patients because otherwise, patients are just spinning their wheels going from one doctor to another, with each telling them something different. Patients in pain are not great advocates for themselves and don't necessarily make the best decisions in that moment. They need to have a cohesive team of health care professionals who are looking out for their best interests and considering all possible modalities to help them.

SPENDING TIME WITH PATIENTS

Doctors who successfully work with CPP patients have the mindset that their patients need to be heard. They will take the time to listen and comfort patients instead of rushing them out the door. Even in the busiest, but effective practices, if the doctor cannot spend sufficient time with patients, she ensures there is a properly trained staff available to do so.

Sandy DiDona, Dr. Echenberg's nurse, said that patients often need a pep talk during their visits and even in-between. Patients often get discouraged when things don't improve quickly, and it helps to remind them of their plan of care. She said, "Sometimes, all they need is someone to talk to, someone who validates their pain, and encourages them to stick to their treatment plan and trust it will work."

DiDona told me that she feels very emotional when working with patients, but she knows it's critical that she stay focused and calm because, "Sometimes we're the only hope they have, and I don't want to lose it when I'm with them.

So I maintain my composure. I give them some sense of security and stability so they know that we're going to be there for them."

Because he is deluged with patients wanting his help, Dr. Steege cannot always spend all the time he knows his patients need and deserve, so he, too, has an exceptionally capable and compassionate nursing staff that can pick up where he must leave off.

> There's a lot of talk and a lot of handholding over the phone. We routinely see three or four new patients in a morning and then six or seven returns. You know, with really challenging new pain problems, we do have to slow down and take an hour, an hour and a quarter because that's time well spent and you lay the groundwork for further work.

DOCTORS NEED TO KNOW THE RIGHT QUESTIONS TO ASK

Asking the right questions is critical for care providers to both diagnose and to refer patients appropriately. As a clinical psychologist and sex therapist, Dr. Judy Kuriansky cannot perform physical examinations. However, she said, "I'm always asking questions, such as: How much does it hurt? How often does it hurt? Does it hurt as much if a finger is inserted? Can you relax, and does that lessen the pain? This last question helps determine the difference between a psychological issue and a physical problem."

Dr. Daniel Brookoff, oncologist and director of the Center for Medical Pain Management at Presbyterian-St. Luke's Medical Center in Denver, Colorado, understands that patients are intimately familiar with their pain. "A lot of doctors don't give you the opportunity to talk to them. It's more important that we *listen* to you than talk to you, because if we give you enough time in a safe place, you will tell us what's wrong. You'll tell us by explaining your pain, whether you have pelvic floor dysfunction or bladder lining dysfunction or fibromyalgia."

Dr. Brookoff insists the doctor must be guided by what the patient says and by a thorough exam to determine if testing is warranted. He explained, "The older you get, you realize that testing is just to confirm what you were thinking anyway. Once in a while, you get surprised. But when you look back on it, the patient was always trying to tell you. Some people have been really tossed around and they've got a million things wrong with them, and everybody tells them they're nuts because there's not just one thing wrong." But Dr. Brookoff is certain that if the practitioner is educated in CPP and listens to his patient, he will eventually learn the whole story.

So Dr. Brookoff can help patients uncover vital pieces of their history they aren't even aware will help him help them. For instance, he said, "Maybe their whole family had the problem or they had symptoms since they were a child.

There are other issues, like a history of abuse, which need to be accounted for. It should be done up front and it shows respect for the person's life. It saves time in the long run because I'm not going to learn much about you in 10 minutes."

PATIENTS DESERVE TO BE HEARD

Once he left his OB practice, Dr. Perry was able to spend the amount of time with his patients he knew they needed. He created a schedule that would meet that need instead of focusing on how many patients he could see in a day. He said, "I decided that I would allot 30 to 45 minutes for every new pain patient and I wouldn't take more than three or four a day. So, sometimes you can do one in 30 minutes, sometimes it takes an hour and a half. But that's the way I wanted my practice to go."

According to Dr. Brookoff, if he gives you two hours up front, then there's more likelihood that he can diagnose you and help you get better more quickly. But if he doesn't spend the time up front, he'll spend a lot more time overall learning in little bits. He said, "I think it's worth putting in the time up front, and I think everybody deserves the opportunity to tell you their whole story, uninterrupted. At least once. And then you have a real basis to go by."

Dr. Lyndsay Elliott, clinical psychologist, is highly skilled in a wide variety of techniques and tailors treatment to each patient:

> I don't go off my own protocol. I'm not in the patient's body. I don't know her symptoms, triggers, psychological issues, or relationships. It's so complex and the patient and I have to work together to figure it out. Sometimes it's hard for patients to tolerate that it's going to take some time and that they can't come into my office and I'm going to fix them in six sessions. It really, really, really takes some time.

She also subscribes to the philosophy that the patient has to be an active partner with her in dealing with core issues. She said, "If they haven't resolved some of their integrative, long-term, deeply painful psychological issues, no behavioral technique I give them is ever really going to sustain them for any significant amount of time."

PARTNERING WITH PATIENTS

An effective CPP practitioner exhibits a caring attitude and validates the patient's experience. In addition, these physicians and their staff want patients to give them honest feedback and are open to learning new information from them.

During the first visit with a patient, Dr. Kahn ensures he covers the two most important issues when beginning a successful treatment plan for CPP.

First, he said that he acknowledges the patient's pain. Second, he tells the patient that she must be a partner on this journey.

Because of his expertise in diagnosis and treatment of patients, Dr. Kahn said, "I can put an individualized plan together quickly. But I like to work with my patients as a team. I'm not just writing them prescriptions and sending them on their way. I want the patient to be involved in managing the problem."

PATIENT COMPLIANCE IS VITAL

Even the best and most caring doctor cannot heal the patient alone. Chronic conditions, as we've seen, are complex and take time to unravel. We live in a society where we demand magic bullets. That's what we expect. Give me a pill to make me feel better—instantly!

That's just not possible with chronic pain conditions such as CPP. First, you have to diagnose all the interrelated parts, then develop a treatment plan that may have to shift as you go through it, and finally, give it all time to work. It's clear from the stories of women and men whose lives and relationships have improved that they work hard to effect the change. Chronic conditions take years to fester and develop. Healing them, especially when they are diagnosed after so much damage, takes time, time, time—and a lot of effort.

While the doctor must do his or her part, investing time, energy, and expertise to help restore the patient's quality of life, so must the patient be willing to do the hard work as well. Often, multiple types of treatment are required to reduce flare-ups, so if the patient is not vigilant, the simmering symptoms are waiting in the wings doing push-ups.

But DiDona, Dr. Echenberg's nurse, also understands the other side as to why some women are less compliant than others are, and it has to do with trust and negative experiences with the medical community. She said:

> Some women balk at the list of medications we recommend that would be helpful for them along with all other modalities. They don't want to take any medication. They're afraid of everything.
>
> Either they've been given some of these medications in higher doses than is called for, or they've been given shotgun by different doctors, a little bit of this and a little bit of that. Then, nothing is working and these chemically sensitive women are just left with side effects and no relief.

EDUCATING PATIENTS

Dr. Kahn is adamant that his patients become educated in their condition. When they leave after their first visit, he'll have them go to certain Web sites to read up on the diagnosed condition. He said, "She'll understand a little bit and read a little bit about what I think will help her. And then, we create her treatment plan together."

KIM'S STORY: 10 YEARS OF PAIN FINALLY LED TO RELIEF

Kim is 26 years old and has been diagnosed with IC and CPP. Ten years earlier, at 16, she was already sexually active and experienced pain during intercourse, as well as heavy bleeding and clots during menstruation. Her pelvic pain quickly became a constant companion.

Based on the advice of a close friend who had endometriosis, Kim saw a gynecologist and asked for a laparoscopy to confirm the diagnosis. She said, "The first doctor told me I was too young for the procedure and that I should have a baby and all my pain would go away. I thought, 'Did this lady actually just tell me to have a baby at 16 years old?' I was very confused, so I started to do some research on my own and found that I did have a lot of symptoms that could be linked to endometriosis."

She found another doctor who performed the laparoscopy and Kim was diagnosed with endometriosis. She was both relieved and excited at the prospect of finally getting rid of her pain. However, she was very wrong.

> I've seen seven doctors and had four laparoscopies. Every doctor said my pain was from the endometriosis and that I just had to learn to cope with the pain. They kept doing surgery [attempts to remove endometriosis implants], only to tell me that the lesions grew back from the last time I had surgery and they would extract them again. I got so sick and tired of hearing the same thing over and over, and not finding anyone who could help me deal with the pain. One doctor actually told me that it was all in my head and gave me a prescription for Zoloft!

Kim was fed up. She was 21 and tired of all the invasive procedures, so she found a doctor who put her on birth control pills, which controlled the daily pain by limiting her periods to four that year. However, intercourse became intolerably painful. She asked her doctor about it and was told, "Well, try different positions," or "you'll just have to deal with it because of the endometriosis." Kim said, "I felt hopeless. No one should have to endure pain like this."

Four years later, she happened to see a sign for a conference at her college titled "Women's Chronic Pelvic Pain and Sexual Disorders." She went to the conference, where Dr. Echenberg was speaking, and said, "I was on my way to recovery."

Within a few days, she became a patient. Dr. Echenberg put her on a comprehensive treatment plan to address all of the issues that caused her pain. The other doctors she'd seen didn't understand the interrelationship between the various systems and organs in the body that converge to cause CPP. Not only did Dr. Echenberg treat her illness, but like all of the doctors I've interviewed who effectively work with CPP patients, he educated her as well. Kim explained:

> Dr. Echenberg taught me that all of the muscles are interconnected in the pelvic floor, and that the bladder and all the other organs are so close to each other that he treats everything at the same time. I never had a doctor explain why so many things were going on with my body and that they could all be treated. I was ecstatic. I was at the point in my life where this was the last straw and if this didn't work, I guessed I would just have to deal with it with no hope of getting better. It is now November 7, 2008, and I am feeling the best I've ever felt in my entire life.

PATIENTS NEED A QUARTERBACK

According to Dr. Perry, someone must be in charge of managing the patient. He said, "It's far too much stress in just dealing with the day-to-day pain for the patient to have to figure it out on her own." His philosophy was that one doctor must ensure that patients are not left to fend for themselves if they are sent off to other specialists for treatment:

> You have to use all your weapons and be familiar with them. The gynecologist has to be the quarterback. He should be the one directing the care. And he shouldn't say, "Well, OK. Now I'm sending you to Dr X."
> He should say, "You need to go to Dr X and you need to come back and see me." If you're going to address chronic pelvic pain issues, you have to take long-term responsibility, along with the patient, for their care.

CREATING A NETWORK

Effective pelvic pain specialists, like the late Dr. Perry, must be resourceful but willing to enlist the aid of other specialists when necessary. DiDona agreed and explained that Dr. Echenberg knew his practice had to be different to change his patients' experience with doctors who couldn't or wouldn't help them. He, too, took the initiative to make connections in the pain world with other types of specialists and continued ongoing training to increase, as DiDona said, "The new tricks up his sleeve to help his patients." Like Dr. Perry, when Dr. Echenberg sends patients to other doctors for specialized treatment, the patient returns to him for continued follow-up.

As is clear by now, the new approach to treating CPP involves the patient seeing not just a single doctor who can address all of the many issues involved with this chronic condition, but a network of providers who work as a team to address the specific areas that need treatment. No one doctor can provide treatment for a patient with a complex set of issues causing her CPP. For instance, many doctors swear by pelvic floor physical therapy for certain CPP conditions and need physical therapists skilled in this area for referral.

The ideal way to effectively ensure patients are quickly helped by the network of specialists required to treat the whole gamut of issues that converge to cause sexual/pelvic pain is to create medical centers where all like-minded health care professionals would be located within a single, multi-office location. Dr. Echenberg has developed his own database of health care providers to address specialty issues. He's working toward creating just such a centralized office complex where all these specialists will have offices, so patients do not have to travel for the help they need. As he said, "When I'm working with a patient, I wish I could just have them go down the hall and get the internal massage after treatment." Let's face it, going from here to there to everywhere is simply exhausting for patients. Iacovelli agreed that it's easier to manage patients' needs when providers are located close by. "After all," she said, "in a hospital setting, when you have a stroke, you can get the whole team together because they're all at the hospital."

Dr. Nel Gerig, urologist, is working with her hospital administrators to help build her dream of developing such a multidisciplinary pelvic pain clinic.

> We're going to write the grant to get the funding to enable us to do the research to figure out who needs an MRI, who needs diagnostic laparoscopy, who needs urodynamics, who needs physical therapy. And then we're going to develop a true protocol and train every urology and gynecology resident in pelvic pain. This is my career goal.

Experts, such as Dr. Steege, agree that referrals work both ways to ensure patients receive the best treatment available. He is fully invested in the patient's quickest and best road to improved health. He said he prefers all doctors learn to recognize which type of specialist is best suited to the patient's particular symptom.

So, for example, if the referring doctor can send patients directly to a pelvic floor physical therapist instead of her sending patients to him first, he said, "The physical therapist and the doctor would work together, which is just fine. There are fewer steps." Rather than feeling concerned that he would be losing patients, Dr. Steege expressed gratitude at the idea of doctors working in this manner, saying, "There are tons of people who need help. I'm not running short of patients."

TENACITY

Dr. Brookoff has a mantra: His patients will get better. He said, "I believe that everyone can get better. But if a doctor offers you a treatment, he or she owes you an expectation. And if the treatment doesn't meet the expectation, it's wrong." But Dr. Brookoff believes that the doctor must have an open mind and keep trying. He said, "Never take no for an answer."

SEE PATIENTS EARLY

According to Dr. Perry, the best chance for success in helping patients recover from CPP is to see patients "fairly early in the process." He believed that
the condition could then more likely be "controlled and reversed." Following
that, patients are ideally sent back to their OB/GYN for routine care. Dr. Echenberg agreed, saying, "The earlier patients see us during the course of their
chronic illness, the quicker they respond and stay improved and can actually
be discharged from the program."

Recognizing early signs of pelvic pain can stave off or eliminate future progression into full-blown chronic sexual pain. The earlier the diagnosis, the less
pervasive the illness ultimately. It's a win for patients, a win for doctors, and a
win for the health insurance industry!

FINAL THOUGHTS

Every patient I interviewed who found proper care told me their symptoms were less upsetting because they had an accurate diagnosis and a health
care provider who listened and validated their concerns. They were no longer
blanketed in fear that these insidious symptoms, misdiagnosed or improperly
treated by uneducated doctors, signaled a fatal disease that would be uncovered too late. In the case of pelvic pain, knowledge, indeed, means power.

For many women who have suffered the indignities of insulting health care
providers, help finally came in the form of not only a knowledgeable doctor,
but one who also exhibited compassion, allowed her to vent her feelings, and
validated all her concerns. While they may still suffer with this chronic condition, most of the patients with whom I spoke noted that this one component
has given them back a will to live and added a greater ability to withstand the
pain.

There are excellent doctors who understand how to diagnose a CPP patient
and who to turn to for specialized assistance. These physicians know how to
connect the dots to see the whole picture.

Those who find good care are not the timid patients, those who slink out of
the doctor's office quietly after being told (or berated) that they're imagining
the pain. Determined CPP patients educate themselves and demand to be
heard. These are the patients who won't stop until they find someone willing
to believe them and go the distance to treat them.

Like them, if you are suffering and have not yet found help, don't stop, don't
yield, don't surrender to your misery. There is help out there. Educate yourself
and keep searching until you find a doctor who will work with you, listen to
you, and give you the care and respect you deserve.

Chapter Fifteen

A DISCUSSION OF PELVIC FLOOR PHYSICAL THERAPY

Pelvic floor physical therapy (PT) has been a godsend for me—it's the only thing that reduces the pain. I have never known sex without pain, but I'm getting close.

—Secret Suffering blogger

They told me the muscles in my vagina were like guitar strings that were strung so tight with what has happened that just touching them caused pain. Maybe that's why a lot of pain was going there, and they're trying to relax the muscles in that area. Their theory is by relaxing that muscle area around the vaginal area, they're attempting to get the pain to subside to some degree.

—Survey respondent

I wanted to include a brief section about pelvic floor physical therapy because so many experts consider it a vital component to the treatment of pelvic floor dysfunction and interstitial cystitis (IC), which a large number of chronic pelvic pain (CPP) patients experience. While there aren't enough physical therapists (PTs) performing this important work, more are recognizing the urgent need to do so.

According to Dr. Echenberg, most women who come to see PTs due to pelvic symptoms come in because of "continence management issues where they are losing their urine." With stress and urinary incontinence, the pelvic floor musculature is usually too lax and loose and these women need to tighten up in an effort to keep this from occurring. He explained:

In women with pelvic pain, this is just the opposite. Most of the people with these pain problems are often in spasm and have pelvic floor tension. So what we have to do is loosen them up and relax them. That's a whole different concept, not just philosophically, but actually in how you work on people.

Continence management centers try to work to tighten women up, for instance, teaching them Kegel exercises, which make some types of pelvic pain much worse. They are addressing the continence, but not dealing with the pain issues. There are a lot of people who have urgency incontinence *and* pain. For those people, Kegels actually make them worse initially. Ultimately, a good pelvic floor PT will find a proper balance of muscle tone for each individual patient.

Sometimes, the pain is too great, and the patient doesn't want to continue PT or to see it through until they experience relief. For the vast majority of CPP patients with pelvic floor dysfunction, however, this therapy has provided amazing relief. Over a few sessions, I learned to tell the difference between the vestibulitis and vaginal (pelvic floor) trigger point burning, but it's very subtle. Dr. Nel Gerig, urologist, mentioned the American Physical Therapy Association (APTA) as a possible source for finding a women's health physical therapist in your region who addresses pelvic floor issues.

Jane didn't continue pelvic floor physical therapy very long. She said, "It made me worse. Yeah, she found my trigger points and she *triggered 'em.*" She knew that Dr. Echenberg was a proponent of physical therapy, but, she said, "When I said it made me worse and I tense up just thinking about it and this is not for me, he said 'Ok, well let's take that off the program and see what else we can do.' He's good about working with his patients and listening to them."

Here is where the advocate for the patient, the gynecologist or other lead doctor, can make a big difference by listening to the patient and having a multimodality approach to the problem and an arsenal of weapons. Whipping chronic pain patients into shape is never the answer. Perhaps Jane would have eventually benefited from PT, but the increased pain from the initial sessions was too much for her.

LIVING WITH CPP: SUSAN'S JOURNAL

My own experience with a pelvic floor physical therapist was very odd to me, too intimate for my comfort—but extremely useful. My own physical therapist and other PTs with whom I spoke said that when people disappear, they really don't know why, but the weirdness I experienced may account for some of the dropout rate.

First, let me say that I felt lucky to have found a PT in Florida who performs pelvic floor physical therapy and has treated IC and sexual pain patients for years. She also treats any kind of chronic and acute pain, as all PTs do. She was a consummate professional.

She works in a podiatrist's office, in the back room, which was kind of funny to me. All these seniors getting their calluses shaved and their ingrown toenails clipped while my most personal of body parts got poked and massaged. In addition, it seemed an uncomfortable idea to begin with. Someone, a stranger, touching me down there and actually using her fingers to press on painful trigger points to release them, just like in my shoulder, only in my vagina. Not to mention, I've heard that these specialized PTs sometimes use a dilator, which is, to me, just another name for a dildo, raising my anxiety level even higher.

However, I've been interviewing PT specialists for this book, and they are all dedicated women passionate about helping other women find long-lasting relief from their pain and very serious when discussing their work. So, I went to see the PT. The first session lasted two hours, and I ended up feeling very comfortable with her. Plus, the loud whirring of the callous remover in the next room was somehow soothing and reassuring. Of course, I was still fully clothed and all of the treatment still theoretical.

She first checked out my back. Then she had me sit on her hand and pressed some points in my back. I was astonished to feel the pain *in my back* radiate directly into my pelvis! She really worked the trigger points on my back, and the pain subsided. Amazing. I felt comforted.

Then, she hooked me up to this biofeedback machine and had me do Kegels, which showed my pelvis was completely tight. In fact, I was nearly off the charts lying still. (After working on me, by the way, my pelvis returned to nearly a normal relaxed level.)

Off came my pants and she had me lie spread-eagle on the table, naked from the waist down. She was chatting with me as we began. I'm no prude and I'm not shy, but my comfort zone was decreasing rapidly.

In she went and pressed on the exact areas where the pain during intercourse made me want to run screaming out of the room, never to let my husband come near me again. When I asked how she found these points, she told me that they feel like nodules of varying types and size. Eventually, some of the points were relieved. The first session was overwhelming, but I was a believer.

For the second session, I was more relaxed walking in. Pretty quickly I was on the table, and here's where the trouble began. I can only speak for myself, but I was there to find relief not only for my day-to-day living, but so I could have pain-free intercourse with my husband. I no longer want to feel like there are hot pokers and burning sandpaper and knives tearing me to bits when he is inside of me. So, the point was to have my vagina feel good, right? This time, the points released more, and she could dig deeper inside my body. A few times it felt like her arm was touching my clitoris. And I nearly shouted at her to move her arm away. I was unnerved.

It felt good. Sexual sensations welled up inside of me. I totally tensed up fearing I would have an orgasm right on the table.

The PT did nothing wrong. Nothing different from the last session.

I freaked out. A lot. I felt like I was cheating on my husband. However, what I have learned through years of recovery from food addiction is that to keep such things a secret, not to talk about them, is the worst thing I can do. But I was sure not going back to see her.

I finally talked to my husband. Just flat out said that it felt too good. Then, I asked him to go with me and learn how to do this to me, himself. My husband wasn't willing. He wouldn't even consider the idea of learning how to do therapeutic trigger point therapy at the PT's office, despite the fact that his fingers have often done the walking along that territory in the bedroom.

He said the PT is a professional and I should discuss it with her, and if I feel those sensations, not to panic because it's part of the treatment. In fact, he said it was OK if I had an orgasm right there on the table because it was therapy! I was aghast, pretty well horrified. Apparently, he wasn't afraid of my running off with the PT, but I tend to think it was more his own anxiety and embarrassment about hands-on training in front of the PT.

I spoke to Dr. Echenberg and to some of the other experts. I asked them if anyone had ever mentioned this as a factor, and they all said no. Either other women simply weren't talking about it, or they weren't experiencing such things, and I was the only one who ever felt this way. Well, that sucked.

Lisa Iacovelli, the physical therapist I interviewed, said, "I've questioned it myself, and thought that, of course one would feel that sensation. I'm aware of that when I'm treating patients. In my practice, women of all ages have felt comfortable with me. Of course, I've had people who disappear and I would imagine that at times they did have those feelings."

However, Dr. Echenberg echoed exactly what my husband said, which annoyed me to no end. He absolutely felt it was OK to feel these sensations. He told me that I needed to go back and talk to her about my feelings.

When I went back to my PT's office, I sat down and immediately burst into a long-winded, run-on sentence, emotional outburst that lasted about five minutes. Her reaction was interesting. She laughed. She wasn't insulted. She was kind and understanding. For one thing, she said she'd also never had anyone tell her that, which made her wonder as well about patients who stopped treatment, because they wouldn't necessarily give her an explanation. For another, she showed me the notes she sent to my doctor and pointed out that when I asked her to move her arm she had been leaning on the perineum, not touching my clitoris at all. This just told me how out of touch with my body I was.

We talked through it for over an hour, and I felt much, much better about it all. So we had our third session. But this time, we worked on my shoulder.

A few weeks went by. I still couldn't deal with a woman putting her fingers inside of my vagina. Especially in the back of the podiatrist's office. This was ridiculous because she just wanted me to feel better, but for me, feeling better felt worse in this context.

I tried using my own fingers, but getting to those deep muscles made me feel like a contortionist, which was definitely *not* a sexual turn-on, and caused me to tense my muscles even more. I begged my husband to learn to do this. At first, he absolutely refused, despite my seductive comment about how it would vastly improve our sex life. He still reacted with a look of horror on his face.

Then one night, after my circus act of trying to get my fingers in there, I begged him again. He commented to no one in particular after a long sigh, "I'm too old for this."

I offered him gloves, so he wouldn't feel weird. "Gloves," he said, "I don't need those, my fingers have been in there before." So I got into position and talked him through it. Amazingly, he found one of the trigger points and I talked him through how to press, while I pushed on my leg as the PT taught me. I stopped him after about three minutes. He was astonished at the level of pain I experienced because he said he had hardly pressed on it. I praised him to the rafters, which works like a charm with this particular man to encourage a repeat of behavior (Pavlov comes to mind). I told him we'd only need to do this three times a week.

I felt buoyant and hopeful that maybe help was finally on the way. Two hours later, he longed for sex. I guess it worked to stimulate something between us. So that night, we shared intimacy, shared an orgasm, shared our lives, and I was able to say no to the pain of intercourse because for that night, he got it. Unfortunately, we both became lazy and didn't really keep up the treatment.

I was still determined to follow through with my physical therapy, and I had gone through three more sessions. Each time, there were points where her hand touched places that turned me on. I had to work hard at not allowing myself to feel those feelings. Clearly, there is no way to have fingers moving around down there without a sexual component. But I have to say that I was improved in some ways, though my bladder symptoms had severely flared. The burning at her touch subsided. Places she could barely touch a few sessions back she was now able to deeply move her fingers into the muscle. From my own experiences with trigger points on my back and shoulders, these are just more trigger points, and the release is similar in feeling.

One physical therapist I interviewed told me about this little gizmo called the Crystal Wand that can reach the inner vaginal muscles to massage them. For want of a better phrase, it's a curved dildo with a strange round ball on one end, and the other end is curved with a slightly rounded point on the end. She trains her patients to use it at home (the curved end). Just to let you know, it's also supposed to be able to reach the G-spot. Of course, that would assume you've massaged the pain out of those trigger points first because G-spot or not, it isn't going to feel good if it hurts.

So I bought the wand and asked my PT to help me learn how to use it. And it works. But you have to be careful not to press too hard, or as I did, you may get cramps. The only other problem is that you can feel the burning with it, but it's not easy to feel the knots or the throbbing or heat as the knots release.

She also gave me some other exercises to take with me, exercises to do fully clothed. These are ways to stretch out the muscles of the pelvis, just like she gave me some exercises to stretch out my back and shoulder.

I talked to Dr. John F. Steege, gynecologist and professor and chief of the Advanced Laparoscopy and Pelvic Pain division, Department of Obstetrics and Gynecology at the University of North Carolina at Chapel Hill, about my experience and got my courage up to describe my feelings. It was a little odd to do so. After all, here is a highly venerated expert. But how would I know my experiences were uniquely neurotic if I didn't keep asking experts if any of their own patients had a similar experience? He said:

> So far there are some women who simply won't go if they're not comfortable with the idea of transvaginal work. We tell them ahead of time, "This is not like having a pelvic exam. This is how they are trained to work."
>
> I do think it is an issue for some people, although generally speaking, the PTs who are good at this are good enough that they work past it and it becomes a non-issue after a while. These PTs develop a level of trust with the patient that serves that relationship well.

I felt relieved by his sentiments. Clearly, as Dr. Steege confirmed, physical therapy is one of the keys to pelvic pain treatment. But still, it was nice to know that I wasn't the only one who experienced an emotional discomfort. And his validation of my experience put me even more at ease about it. Ultimately, I discovered a lot of people with whom I spoke felt a little odd about this physical therapy at first, but those who stuck with it got past their discomfort when they began to get lasting relief.

A SPOUSE'S POINT OF VIEW

I posted my experiences on the *Secret Suffering* Web site, and shortly thereafter, I received a posting in response. I have reprinted it in its entirety.

> I am the spouse of a woman that, except for your food allergies, has a list of maladies very similar to yours. Her problems began in her mid-twenties. It is now 30 years later. Over the last year she has gone through the therapy you are describing. Once the situation started to improve, I was asked to go and learn the techniques because the treatments are needed more than once or twice a week. It felt weird having a young woman telling and showing me what to do, demonstrating on my wife what I'm supposed to be feeling for and the proper way to apply the pressure and when,

where, and how to palpate the areas for the most effective results. But remember, the purpose of all of this was to achieve a reduced pain, if not outright pain free, existence for my wife. And IT WORKS!

There are lots of nerves and receptors in that region of your body. The first few times you will be learning the sensations as well as receiving a treatment. It has been almost a year since we started down this path and we still find something new every once in a while.

There are a couple of things you have to decide. The first seems rather simple, but in our society it is not. The treatment is not a sexual act. The treatment is partially performed on the part of your body that is used for sexual activity. But there is a huge difference.

The second is your approach to the treatments. The purpose of the treatment is to improve your health. You have to be comfortable with the therapist and the setting. The treatments should always be private. The only time someone else should be in the room is if they are receiving instruction (your significant other) or they are necessary for the treatment itself (to help you position yourself, to monitor equipment, etc.) or another medical professional for consultation purposes related to your condition. And you have to actually converse with your therapist about what is going on.

This isn't something being done to you. You are a participant. If an entire treatment session is spent just discussing what is going on with the recommended course of treatment that is time well spent. I'm sure you are somewhat tense. After all, someone is messing in places that "aren't supposed to be messed with." Your tension is something that contributes to the problem. It is a vicious cycle. Have your therapist discuss the cycle of pain. That is what you are trying to break.

One thing to remember, there are times and certain trigger points that will actually cause referred discomfort (OK, out and out pain). The pain will usually start to subside during the treatment or a short time afterward.

Since a lot of the problems are related to tension, plan a quiet period after a treatment. Perhaps even with a warm towel or pillow on your lower abdomen. A 15 or 30 minute nap is not inappropriate.

Please go back to the therapist. Get over the sexual feelings. By that I mean quit worrying about it. The fact that your body responds to the relief of pain and enjoys the stimulation is fantastic. It means there is hope for you to enjoy that side of your life again. Your body's response has nothing to do with the gender of the person providing the relief. It is your body enjoying the relief! As long as you and your therapist keep it professional, there is no problem. Even if you do experience an orgasm.

Please try to convince your spouse to go with you and learn the techniques. After all, he would probably give you a back rub if you asked. This is really no different. My wife was afraid that I'd be grossed out by what might be required. That may be part of your significant other's concern. In many ways it is like caring for an infant. It isn't gross. It isn't dirty. It is a task that is necessary and like taking care of a baby, it is done with gentleness and the proper level of attention. But one does have to learn the proper way to do the treatments. And the only way to do that is with hands-on training under the guidance of a professional that knows what to look for and how to treat the problems. And yes, that took some getting used to for me.

You may find out that once the pressure points (or trigger points) have been backed down from their highly inflamed state that the treatment may become part of your foreplay because it helps ensure that there isn't any pain during sex.

This therapy gave me back the woman I married over 35 years ago. She can walk without pain, and without crutches or a cane. Something she hasn't been able to do for over 10 years. While her brothers and sisters (and I) are complaining about the aches and pains of growing of older, she revels in being able to do ordinary, everyday chores without chronic pain.

Please try again. Patience, persistence, and commitment will help.

Chapter Sixteen

AMY: THE HIGH VALUE OF INTIMACY FOR A CANCER SURVIVOR

Amy, who's in her mid-40s, lives with a myriad of health challenges. Not only does she suffer with chronic pelvic pain (CPP) and interstitial cystitis (IC), she has recovered from breast cancer and thyroid tumors as well as the removal of her ovaries. In addition, in her late teens, she was raped and beaten by an ex-boyfriend, an imprinting of her nervous system that may well have contributed to her CPP.

When I arrived for our interview, I met an upbeat, warm woman who looked the picture of health, with glowing bronzed skin and shiny, chin-length blonde hair. You'd never know by looking at her just how tortured her body and soul have been because of all she's suffered. In fact, she said, "When I took a fibromyalgia quiz recently, 8 out of 10 of my answers were positive indicators of the condition. But I think I'm like most women with these problems. Doctors just tell us to deal with them."

Amy, the mother of two teen boys, loves kids and "the wonderment and magic of childhood. I've just never grown up. I won't." She was a sixth grade teacher for learning-disabled children until she was diagnosed with breast cancer. Her husband, Martin, designs cars.

Amy constantly suffered with bladder infections throughout her teens, which caused her to have severe depression. But when she was 16, she fell in love, and at 17, she had intercourse. "It was absolutely, wretchedly horrible. I hated it from day one," she said. "It was like someone had just taken a hot poker to me."

At first, Amy thought the pain was normal for a girl experiencing sex for the first time. She was fully educated about sex by a mother who wanted to ensure her daughters would not naïvely walk through the world, as she explained:

> My mother always made sure that my sister and I understood our bodies. She was very open about it. She wanted us to know our options as women and how to take care of ourselves to make sure we didn't end up in a bad relationship.

Naturally, Amy didn't tell her mother about her first sexual experience, but she did see a gynecologist about the agonizing pain she'd suffered. Unfortunately, the doctor validated Amy's own incorrect conclusion. "My gynecologist said that sometimes in the beginning, it is quite painful," she told me. But that did nothing to remedy her situation.

> After a while I said, "Something's just not right." I never had an orgasm. I didn't like sex. I didn't want to be touched. But I was in love with this boy. I was confused.
> I enjoyed being with my boyfriend. I didn't have intimacy issues. I didn't blame my father for leaving my mother—didn't carry baggage like that. So I couldn't understand why it hurt so much physically.

Suddenly, without warning, the relationship turned violent. After two years, her boyfriend began beating her. She broke up with him. And then, he raped her. Amy described what happened:

> He watched my house. He knew my schedule. He waited until my mother was gone for a week. Then he broke into the house, held a knife to my neck, and said, "I know your mother's gone. If you make a peep, I know your sister's in the next room. I'll cut her up."

She said that, because she knew him, it was just easier to lie there than resist the violent assault. She said, "Unfortunately, I was the dumb victim who thought that if she would have done something differently, this wouldn't have happened. He wasn't a stranger on the street. He hadn't been violent like that. So I just lay there. I took it. And finally he left."

At the time, Amy didn't want anyone to know what happened. But being the strong woman that she is, she dealt with this assault in her own way. "I wrote him a nasty note. Then I went to his prized, expensive sports car, and took a solid metal baseball bat to it. I left the note, which said, 'If you have any contact with me in the future, I will tell my dad.' And that was enough. I didn't see or hear from him again. But it took a long time for me to be intimate again. A long time."

When Amy finally got involved in another relationship a year later, it took eight months after they met for her to have sex with him:

My boyfriend was very patient. He was wonderful, but I had never had an orgasm with intercourse. I didn't know what it felt like. I was still waiting for this wonderful thing to happen. But he was about nine inches long—huge! It was painful! It was horrible! Because he understood how much intercourse hurt, he was very gentle and kind. And he would always satisfy me afterward.

LIVING WITH CPP: SUSAN'S JOURNAL

I've always been mystified by the mysterious and elusive (for me anyway) intercourse orgasm. Even though volumes have been written on how to accomplish this marvelous feat, I feel lucky to have *any* orgasm.

It's like when I had the C-section and felt embarrassed that I couldn't give birth naturally. I felt less than a woman. Finally, someone sensible asked, "Isn't the point to have the baby? Does it really make you more or less of a woman how it comes out?"

I personally feel the same way about orgasms, though I must admit to having my moments during the act where it was close, really, really close, and just like in the Kentucky Derby, I wanted my horse to finish first. But after 53 years on this planet, no luck. So I'm just grateful to achieve the final result any way I can.

AMY'S AMBIVALENCE

I told Amy I knew only two women who had orgasms with intercourse and wondered if she thought she was abnormal for not being able to do so. She responded, "Yes, I thought most people did. I didn't get it. I didn't think it was unrealistic to hope for one every now and then."

Like many, Amy equated intercourse with sex. I asked her what she would do when intercourse hurt.

> I'd just grit my teeth and bear it. I don't think my boyfriend knew it hurt. I was afraid if I told him he would leave. I was very afraid of jeopardizing the relationship. I was head over heels in love. And I could see myself spending the rest of my life with him.
>
> Again, I think it was because I was so young. I was 20. And I wasn't a career girl. I mean, yeah, I was going to college and I was probably going to be a history teacher, but for me it was about getting married and having kids. All I've ever wanted was to be a mom.

Despite her continued willingness to endure painful intercourse with the man she loved, her relationship ended after she discovered he'd been cheating on her. Ironically, she said the cheating wasn't because of any sexual issues between them but because she was working three jobs to put herself through college and only saw him on Friday nights.

Her boyfriend's best friend was the one who told her. Amy was devastated. She had tried so hard to do everything right—paying her way through college at age 21 and being a loyal girlfriend. "I became so depressed I debated ending my life," she admitted. "But then I realized how dumb it was to end my life for someone else. I looked at myself in the mirror and said, 'You have to snap out of this. It's got to end.'"

This part of Amy's story has a happy ending. She and her ex-boyfriend's best friend became close, developed a strong friendship, and fell in love. The best friend is now Amy's husband, Martin. Unlike her previous relationship, Amy was completely honest and told Martin the truth about her CPP long before they were sexually involved. "That's how I knew Martin was the right person, because I told him everything from day one. Nothing was hidden."

Their friendship continued for a year before it became romantic. She described the transition from a platonic to sexual relationship:

> We had sex on our first serious date, one year after we became romantically involved. It was uncomfortable. We weren't very good together in the beginning. But he's never been rough. He's always been a very gentle man and lover. Since he knew from the beginning that I hated sex, and couldn't orgasm with intercourse, he took the time to ask questions and find out what felt good. And when he knew it was uncomfortable, he was careful.

Amy felt responsible for her illness interfering with sex, but she found ways around the pain. She realized that if she had an orgasm before intercourse, her pelvic muscles tightened. She didn't know how to relax them at that time, though she's since learned to do so through physical therapy. So it was easier for her to let Martin penetrate her after a lot of foreplay and have his own orgasm before bringing her to orgasm.

Sometimes, depending on the position during intercourse, Amy would still find it too painful. But she learned to keep it simple. She said, "Let's face it: if you analyze the whole thing to death while you're doing it, sex isn't much fun. If I hurt, it was easy enough to say, 'Can we try another position?' Or, 'Can you give me a minute?'"

Before they got married, Amy and Martin had sex whenever they saw each other, probably once a week. After moving in together, and to this day, they have sex two to three times a week.

Amy grew up having a lot of urinary tract infections but didn't suspect that her sexual pain was bladder-related. Gynecologists continually dismissed her problems. Amy finally resigned herself to trusting that the doctors were right. After all, they'd been to medical school. At least three gynecologists told her the pain was due to the way she was built and the fact that she'd had kids. She decided to deal with it, accepting that it was just plain painful for some people.

I'd tell the doctors certain positions hurt and they'd tell me, "Don't do them." Well, duh! But you can't always lie there missionary style. There's got to be some spice in the relationship, you know? The way to keep a marriage healthy is to keep it spicy. Your wife shouldn't lie there, like a board, with her eyes closed saying, "Please just get it over with." How fun is that for a guy?

Despite her incessant attempts at a positive outlook in the face of pain, Martin knew when Amy hurt. His response was, "I'll try to be as fast as possible." About this consideration, she said, "He was very understanding, and sometimes I'd do it if he was in the mood and I wasn't. I think it's one of those give and takes. I think that's also part of being intimate. But I didn't lie to him."

As our interview went on, I became more curious about this. A supportive husband. A woman who hurts. Didn't he ever say, "Honey, let's stop if it hurts you?" Amy answered:

What he would say is, "Can I change the angle for you? Can I try another position for you?" Sometimes he would just stimulate me manually for a few minutes while he was inside of me so he could finish, even though it was very difficult for me to orgasm that way.

Based on her husband's shifting-position attitude—to keep on truckin' rather than withdraw—I asked Amy if he was one of those men who considered intercourse the be all and end all of sex? Adamantly not. "Oh, no. He doesn't care how we have sex. Again, he's known from day one. He's really easygoing. This is nothing new. We've been together almost 20 years."

How perplexing to me to hear this last statement in light of all her previous comments about she and Martin's sex life. I wasn't sure now if she was the one insistent on including intercourse no matter the price because of her guilt or desire, or if she knew or he told her how important it was to him to have intercourse, despite her last statement.

Amy gave birth to her children in her late 20s and found it especially painful having sex when pregnant. She said, "I guess it was because of the way I was carrying the babies. It seemed like they all sat on my bladder. After each of my children was born, I had terrible, flaming urinary tract and yeast infections."

These bladder episodes came on suddenly and violently without warning, between one normal trip to the bathroom and an abnormal trip when she'd bleed and hurt. She described the experience this way:

The urgency was terrible, and the burning hellacious. I felt like my bladder was so full that if I didn't go, I was going to lose it. I could stay on the potty a long time and the urgency just wouldn't go away. I used to carry urine cups with me so that when I flared up, I always had a cup to take into my doctor's office. They could just dip a stick, give me medication, and I'd be on my way.

But her doctors at the time continued insisting the pain was all in her head. Although she was angry about that, she said, "You get used to it, plus I'm a person who believes everything in your life is there for a reason. As freaky as that sounds, maybe the pain was telling me that I needed to be with Martin because he was the first one who understood my pain."

When Amy was in her early 30s, her husband inadvertently discovered a lump in her breast during sex. She said, "He went to move his arm and bumped me under my breast. It felt as if he had stabbed me! When we were finished, I got up, felt it, and thought, 'Oh my God. I have something there. OK. Don't panic.' I knew the first thing they'd ask is if I have breast cancer in my family, which I don't."

Even with something as serious and potentially deadly as breast cancer, Amy found that doctors were dismissive and difficult. But she had already learned to be her own advocate. On the phone, her gynecologist said it sounded like the lump was an inflamed milk duct. Amy didn't think so. Her suspicions had grown stronger, despite the lack of breast cancer in her family history. That afternoon, she saw her family doctor and insisted on receiving a sonogram that day. The sonographer was patronizing, saying, "Lady, it's a cyst; go home."

The next week, Amy saw a breast surgeon who biopsied the area. Amy said, "He pulled out the syringe filled with this black pudding." Cancer. She had a lumpectomy the next week. The doctor assured her she had clean margins, meaning the cancer was contained and they had removed it all. But he was wrong. The cancer turned out to be severely aggressive. Within four months, she discovered three more lumps. The cancer was progesterone receptor positive, which meant that the lumps grew during her period.

Before her next period, she had a double mastectomy. "It was almost exactly two months from the day I found the lump until the day the breasts were off. I wasn't fooling with it. The doctor didn't want to do the surgery. He said I had clean margins. I was young, healthy, no history. He wouldn't touch a thing. But I found another surgeon who listened to me."

Amy's gut told her the same thing when it came to her CPP. She no longer believes that the doctor is automatically right simply because he acts like an authority figure. "If a doctor tells you something, check all your options. I mean, yes, you do have to trust the doctor to a certain extent, but you have to trust *yourself* first."

Amy said her husband completely supported her decision to have a radical mastectomy:

> Martin didn't care. He just wanted the cancer gone. He said, "You do whatever you need to do to get well. Let's get you healthy. I want to keep you around for 50 years."

Most guys would have packed their bags and left. I had such a great support system; it was easy to get healthy. The day my hair fell out due to chemo treatments, my older son shaved his head so he could look like me.

Though Martin is the love of Amy's life, she told him more than once that he should find another woman who doesn't come loaded with the baggage that weighs her down. He consistently responded, "That's not what I want. I love you. I'm with you. This is what I want." About his devotion, she said, "There has never been a doubt in his mind. It's a blessing, especially after the cancer. I mean, good God. I have no breasts and my husband says every day, 'God, you are so hot. You are so cool. I love you. You're the greatest thing.'"

After her surgery, Amy and Martin resumed their sexual life as soon as they were able to do so. "I was taped and bandaged and had drains, and it was about two weeks before we were able to have sex again. Even then it was mostly oral sex. I found it difficult to lie down and have the skin jarred, to have any pressure on me."

But Amy believed having sex was a vital component to normalizing her marriage after all the trauma and to help her husband cope.

I think he needed that reconnection. We slept in separate beds for about three months just because there was so much going on with me. If he rolled onto me, it was terribly painful. I slept with two regular pillows, underarm pillows, and a special head pillow. Plus, I got up every three hours to take pain medication.

She continued on chemotherapy for about six months. Her pelvic pain worsened during that time, the vaginal dryness became severe, and her periods became much more difficult. That made it harder to maintain intimacy in her marriage, but she insists it was an important part of her recovery:

Oral sex was fine, great. That was an easy way to have intimacy and connect. It was very hard psychologically for me to have sex because I felt like I was infecting him . . . like the cancer was everywhere, growing inside of me. I felt disgusting. That's unrealistic and I knew it was unrealistic. He couldn't catch this. I couldn't give it to my kids.

But I still felt like Frankenstein. I had so many freaking scars on me, it was gross. I dressed so he couldn't see the scars. It was easier to think that if he couldn't see the scars, he wouldn't know they were there.

Mostly, it was really important that we get close again. To me, any level of intimacy is a connection, even spooning. It's that time for just the two of us. It doesn't matter if we're holding hands and watching a movie or having intercourse. We're having that time together. So even though it was just oral sex usually, we still experienced orgasms. We still had a connection.

Three years after her treatment for cancer, Amy hit that "magical number when they can stop seeing you every couple of months and test every flipping thing." The doctor convinced her to get genetic testing despite her lack of family history. He thought something was off-kilter about her having such a virulent strain of breast cancer at her age. She tested positive for *BRAC1*. According to Amy, that meant she had an 87 percent chance of breast cancer and an 89 percent chance of ovarian or uterine cancer. This time she had a family history; her aunt had died of ovarian cancer.

A year and a half before this interview, Amy had her ovaries removed. As if this wasn't enough, six months after the ovarian surgery, during a routine dental exam, her dentist felt a swelling on her neck. There were lumps on her thyroid. Amy insisted her oncologist remove her thyroid rather than do a biopsy to see if it was malignant. "My children are still young. I didn't want another phone call with news I'll dread."

While Amy's pelvic pain took a back seat when her health issues were dire, once each crisis had passed, it always resurfaced. She experienced no difference in her level of pelvic pain and still had symptoms of a urinary tract infection about once a year. But miraculously, she finally found help while going to physical therapy for her breasts after her implants. During a session, the therapist asked Amy if she had any pelvic issues. Amy practically screamed with relief. "I just spewed out everything to the therapist." After doing a quick internal exam, she found Amy had serious pelvic issues and referred her to a pelvic pain specialist.

Amy trusted her physical therapist and thought she was brilliant. Because of these treatments, Amy was pain-free in her breast area and was hopeful that finally, she could find relief for her CPP. She went to see the specialist, which she considers a major turning point in her life:

> He told me I had bladder and other pelvic muscle issues, a comprehensive set of problems. He put me on a number of medications, antidepressants, antihistamines, and Elmiron to heal the bladder lining. He wanted to do a series of bladder instillations, but after I finished the fourth one, I was in too much pain. It hurt like hell, worse than the worst UTI I ever had in my life! He also had me shooting creams and gels into my vagina. I began to think it was just not worth all this trouble.
>
> But then one night, Martin and I were having sex and I suddenly realized it didn't hurt! I didn't feel any pain, no urinary symptoms at all. Amazing! And I wasn't even done with the instillation treatments.

AMY'S TREATMENT PROTOCOL

Amy has learned some simple methods to alleviate the pain. She said, "I guess because of my age and all I'd been through, I'd lost my lubrication. I didn't realize that was a problem, but adding additional lubrication during sex helps a whole lot."

One of the first and most important things Amy learned was that doing Kegel exercises—extremely helpful for urinary incontinence—isn't appropriate as a primary method of relaxing the pelvic floor in women who have pelvic floor spasm and pain. Dr. Echenberg said, "Physical therapists, however, do train people to relax certain muscles by first consciously tightening them—very much like biofeedback in which the brain and the vaginal muscles act in harmony rather than dysfunction." Through pelvic floor physical therapy, Amy learned how to recognize and concentrate on relaxing the pelvic muscles before intercourse. This helped her immensely.

Amy is certain that the entire treatment plan, not just one component, was responsible for the miraculous reduction of her pelvic and sexual pain symptoms. She now says the relief she experiences was worth every moment of discomfort during her treatments.

To her relief, after nine weeks, she was finished with the bladder instillations. She certainly didn't enjoy them, but there was no question to her that they vastly increased her ability to have sex. "The instillations got less painful. I still can't say I was very comfortable when I had them, but the nurse would inject a little Lidocaine first, which I think helped to lessen the trauma. And instillations take less than a minute, so I was only in the office about 10 minutes altogether."

Amy has continued using five percent Lidocaine ointment on the vestibular area (just inside the vaginal opening) with good results. "It's absolutely amazing. The first couple weeks, I couldn't feel any pain during sex, but I was so numb, I couldn't orgasm either. Happily, the numbness passed so I could have an orgasm, but I still wouldn't feel the pain." She now uses the Lidocaine on the three days she and Martin have intercourse.

> Every now and then, I'll feel a twinge—definitely if he's penetrating from behind. If I'm not positioned right, my bladder feels a jolt of pain. I cry out, "Oh my God!" and we'll either switch positions or he'll try to change an angle or, just like before, it's easy for me to finish orally. No skin off my back. It's still being intimate.

Amy changed insurance plans and could no longer see her PT. Luckily, she had experienced a lot of relief through their work together, and she began doing exercises at home.

> The PT gave me great stretches to warm up. I vary them so I can get in the pelvic muscles as well as the breasts.
>
> A few weeks ago, for the first time, I was able to jog on the treadmill. I had never been able to do that without a lot of pain and without leaking urine.
>
> Through biofeedback, I've learned to contract the pelvic muscles and build them up. It takes vigilance and it's not fun. It also takes a truckload of time to do all this. I

don't know how a woman who has to work 10 hours a day could do it. I'm lucky I can be sitting at the table doing 20 of my exercises while the kids are having dinner.

Amy has had no major flare-ups since the series of bladder instillations: no infections, no leaking, and just one painful sexual encounter that occurred a few nights before we spoke. "I felt the burning and the stabbing. I think it was just the angle from which he was penetrating. He was just about done—three more thrusts and he was finished."

Amy considers herself a lucky woman, especially after her doctors reassured her about her odds of overcoming the cancer.

> The last thing they were worried about was me dying. But you hear the word *cancer*, and you know it has grown in your body and your cells have formed permutations. The experience has changed the playing field.
>
> I know people who have died from cancer. There's always going to be somebody whose story is worse than yours. Mine wasn't nearly as bad as others. I wasn't given a death sentence.

After all she's gone through, Amy insists that ensuring a strong sexual, intimate connection with her husband is one of the most important components of making her life worth living. She's willing to go to great lengths to keep that connection with her husband. After a mastectomy, chemotherapy, and reconstructive surgery; after having her ovaries and thyroid removed, she's still undergoing treatment for her pelvic pain, saying, "If I could avoid all this crap I would. But I can't, because for those few hours that I'm pain free, I can have sex and have an orgasm, and to me that's everything."

It was fascinating to me that, despite the breadth and depth of Amy's medical issues, continuing to resolve her pelvic pain was of paramount importance to her. Clearly, it struck at the core of what made her life worth living, which was the intimate connection with her husband. It seemed that Amy's attitude exemplified the biological need for couples to connect intimately, with sex, in Amy's case, being the medium of expression. And she was insistent that feeling like a sexual, feminine being has restored her self-esteem, healing many of her emotional scars:

> For Martin and I to have sex, really good sex, and have him roll over and say, "Oh my God. I think that's one of the best things we've ever done," even after being together for 20 years is remarkable to me.
>
> It was huge for me to feel sexy again. I have a new spring in my step. I don't feel like I'm battered and torn. I don't feel so much like Frankenstein anymore. Because of finally having my CPP treated, I have better self-worth and I've learned to listen for the signs of pelvic distress in my body so I can deal with it before it gets out of hand. If I'm sitting on the couch, I can try to be aware of what my pelvis is doing. If my pelvis is tight and knotted, I know how to let go.

Amy advises women with CPP to learn to listen and be aware of your body. "Before you have sex, relax. Take a couple of minutes to massage the vaginal muscles, which a PT can teach you and your partner." Amy continues to follow her own advice before intercourse to have more comfortable sex, such as inserting two or three fingers first and making sure she is lubricated.

Perhaps most importantly, Amy got her wish for that elusive intercourse orgasm. She smiled as she told me, "Three times, to be precise."

AMY'S MESSAGE TO WOMEN WITH CPP

Because of all she's been through, Amy insists that women need to be their own advocate regarding their health. She said, "I think we, as women, forget to take care of ourselves first. When I got cancer, that was my first realization: to stop and take care of myself. But it might take something or someone saying, 'Hey, you need to listen to your body' to become willing to change."

While it's important to remember that CPP doesn't get cured or can't be cut out like a tumor, that doesn't mean you shouldn't find a way to manage your condition. So although sexual/pelvic pain syndrome may not magically disappear even with a treatment plan, Amy believes that every bit of relief increases the quality of life. She is very clear about her message: "Stop being afraid that if you tell somebody something's wrong with your body, there's something wrong with *you*. Please demand the help you deserve!"

SERIES EDITOR AFTERWORD

As we sat in a diner having lunch and talking about her professional future, my student suddenly said that she wanted to share something very personal with me, since it might affect her going through with further graduate studies. She added that she knew I would understand because she was in my class, which addressed issues about relationships, and because I am a psychologist and sex therapist who has talked with innumerable women and men of all ages about very personal issues, including sex.

She proceeded to tell me of her experience of intense pain in very personal sexual parts of her body that had been going on for years and gravely disabled her relationships and every aspect of her life. In fact, at that very moment, she was shifting on the seat in discomfort. She went on to describe the many medical solutions she had pursued, which had failed. She asked me if I would help give public voice to the terrible pain she and many other women were enduring—in silence and shame.

Moved by her sharing, and the egregiousness of the lack of solutions to her suffering, I agreed that I would. I proceeded to research the problem of pelvic pain, by connecting with the National Vulvodynia Association (a nonprofit organization dedicated to educating patients and physicians as well as funding research and providing support groups) and by talking to many women suffering with intense pelvic pain. Intensely moved by their stories, I was particularly enthused when I encountered Susan Bilheimer, who was willing—and keen—to share her personal journey in a book. I knew it would result, as it has, in this excellent book, which includes her personal story and stories of many other women—and men—as well as advice from experts about what to do about what has been a mystery to women and many medical professionals.

Susan's book is hard to put down. Her accounting of her experiences reads as compelling as any novel, except it is that much more powerful and heart-wrenching given that it is real. Fortunately, the horror of the condition is balanced by Susan's honest revelations and helpful tips (64 in all). Further, her connection with her coauthor, Dr. Robert J. Echenberg, an enlightened physician, led to revelations of a multimodal treatment approach to this chronic pain condition. As a result, their book should be in the hands of all women and their partners who suffer from this condition—which a research study reported can affect up to 13 million women, of all ages and in all racial groups.

As a sex therapist for many decades, I know that sex should be pleasurable. And yet, this condition can so gravely interfere with a happy and healthy life, leaving some women unable to exercise, enjoy sex, or even get out of bed. My student told me she couldn't even wear stockings—she cut a hole where the seams in the crotch area are to avoid direct contact.

A beauty queen told me that she gave up her title because of severe pain in her vulvar area. Just sitting on a chair was so unbearable, she had to sit with her legs apart. Pain radiating down her hips made the 34-year-old feel like a 90-year-old.

The pain is so great for some women, they even think of ending their life.

The problem was given some public notice on the TV series *Sex in the City* when the character Charlotte said "my vagina is depressed" and told her gynecologist about vaginal burning, itching, and stinging. The doctor, unfortunately, told her it was not serious, sadly downplaying the devastating impact of the condition.

Despite *Sex in the City* and over 50 years of women's liberation and sex how-to books and media attention, talking about such a disorder "down there" still causes embarrassment and discomfort for the sufferer, their partners, and others hearing about it. It's shocking how little information women and even professionals actually know about this aspect of sexuality, including for example, about words like 'vestibule,' the site of some pain at the entrance to the vagina.

Fortunately, this book explains the physical as well as the emotional and spiritual aspects of this condition, so women—and professionals—*are* informed. *Secret Suffering* provides patients, their partners, and health professionals with invaluable information and advice about what to do about this chronic sexual and pelvic pain. The authors offer a useful scale and questionnaire to pinpoint the problem and solutions that give women support to cope. At the end of reading Susan Bilheimer and Dr. Echenberg's book, there can be no more secrets about this suffering, as the sharing offers invaluable support and help for healing—and loving.

Judy Kuriansky, PhD

Appendix A

SIXTY-FOUR TIPS TO RELIEVE SEXUAL AND PELVIC PAIN*

There are important steps women can take immediately (and some on their own) to help relieve sexual pain and the conditions that cause it. It is imperative that women seek medical help for chronic pelvic pain, but the suggestions that follow can empower women to take charge of their treatment.

Further discussion elaborates on the dangers of products promising "quick fixes" and "magic bullets" that, at best, may not help and, at worst, can be harmful. The use of herbal or topical ointments marketed as an "instant" cure for increasing sexual pleasure may just make the symptoms worse. The use of "natural hormones" or even soy supplements without the direction of a knowledgeable physician may actually create an imbalance if a woman is "estrogen dominant."

The good news is that there are definitely lifestyle changes that will help. For instance, a low-acid diet may help calm vulvar, vaginal, and bladder flare-ups as well as increase bowel health, which is becoming known as an additional trigger for sexual pain. Skin care tips, such as ensuring sexual lubricants, soaps, detergents, and even toilet paper do not contain fragrance, can also make a big difference.

There are many ways women can help themselves while seeking medical assistance to provide more formal, prescriptive methods of treatment. Patience, a willingness to change, and persistence are all ways to begin the path to healing.

*Reprinted with permission from "64 Tips to Relieve Sexual & Pelvic Pain," by Susan Bilheimer with Robert J. Echenberg, MD. Copyright © 2008, Secret Suffering, LLC.

Exercise

1. Be cautious about routine exercises you may already be doing. The pelvic region has many more joints, muscles, and ligaments than you may imagine. Some exercise practices, such as the use of stationary bicycles and stair climbers, may otherwise be very healthy for you. But if you experience sexual pain, these types of exercises might cause extra stress and spasm. "Toning up" may actually be a "sexual downer" on body parts that need to be the most relaxed and comfortable for those intimate moments.

2. Find the softest, most pliable seat possible and wear loose-fitting clothes when riding a bicycle, motorcycle, and even a scooter, or better yet, consider giving up these activities. The pressure against your already-sensitive genital area can cause symptoms to flare up.

3. Give up the attitude of "playing through the pain." While coaches often urge athletes, young and old, to "play through the pain," it's vital to abandon this attitude when it comes to enduring painful sex as an adult. Many women believe that they must have sex to please their partner despite the pain, and if they don't, there's something fundamentally wrong with them. Nothing could be further from the truth. A loving partner would never want to cause such suffering.

4. See a pelvic floor physical therapist. More and more physical therapists (PTs) are incorporating pelvic pain treatment into their practice as the urgency of effectively treating women with sexual pain increases. In fact, a growing number of doctors consider pelvic floor therapy a vital component of a complete treatment plan for sexual pain. Such PTs utilize various methods to release trigger points in the body. Trigger points develop through contraction or spasms in the muscle groups surrounding the vagina, bladder, and lower bowel. Using manual pressure, biofeedback, and other techniques, these health care providers can often aid sufferers in releasing on a physical, emotional, and psychological level. Patients are eventually given exercises to practice at home.

Clothing

5. Wear cotton underwear only, and change it twice a day if possible. Cotton is a more breathable material than silk, polyester, etc., so heat and moisture, both of which are breeding grounds for bacteria, aren't trapped inside. Not sexy? Well, the other half of this admonition is to sleep without underwear at all so your genital area gets to "breathe."

6. Give up wearing thongs. Self-induced "wedgies" can only cause further irritation to those sensitive genital tissues.

7. Realize that tight clothing and pantyhose cause irritation. Many women experience vaginal burning just from wearing fitted jeans. Pantyhose can definitely trap bacteria and tightly press on your genitals. Thigh highs or stockings with a garter belt prevent the problem and can be alluring as well.

Sex

8. Use nonpetroleum, glycerin-free, non–oil-based lubricant products. Astroglide, Femglide, or water-soluble gels such as KY jelly may be good choices. They have no fragrances, colorings, or other ingredients that are common irritants.

9. Try coconut oil. It has a thicker consistency than other single ingredient oils. Coconut oil has proven helpful in enabling sensitive women to experience more comfortable intercourse.

10. Realize that products labeled "gentle" or "natural" can still cause irritation. Baby oil or naturally scented oils may appear to be fine. However, you may still be sensitive to one or more of the ingredients. Most oils for massage, unlike cooking oil, usually have multiple ingredients. Always read the label.

11. Wash your hands before continuing if, during sex, you or your partner has contact with the rectal area (yours or your partner's). If that seems too difficult, be very careful when either of you touch your vulva or vagina afterwards. You may inadvertently contaminate yourself with bacteria, which can lead to an infection. This is true regarding intercourse as well, if there are any residual bacteria on his penis.

12. Consider using dilators to help with certain sexual pain conditions. Dilators are tubes of varying sizes and lengths. Some sex therapists and pelvic floor specialists train patients to use dilators for conditions such as vulvodynia. Similar to a dildo in shape, dilators are used therapeutically to help relax the muscles. Tension is often a learned response to initial pain. When associated with sex, you may unconsciously tighten up in expectation of being hurt. Starting with the smallest size, the patient inserts the dilator as far as is comfortable and is taught to gently squeeze the muscles and then relax. Over multiple sessions, the size of the dilator is increased after the previous size no longer causes any discomfort.

Personal Care

13. Sit on a cushion. Using a cushion or pillow can relieve pressure on your tailbone and genital area when sitting on a hard chair, driving, and so on. There are even specially made cushions for this purpose with cutouts to further reduce the pressure on that sensitive area.

14. Change your pad often. Hormones can change the pH balance of your vagina, especially around your period. This makes you more prone to vaginal infections. Damp pads and blood can cause extreme irritation and also open the way to infection. Change your pad every two hours as a preventive.

15. Use tampons carefully. Tampons soak in far more of the menstrual fluids than pads, allowing for deeper penetration of the irritating fluids and an increased likelihood of infection. Tampon insertion alone can cause a lot of pain when the vaginal tissue is already inflamed or raw.

16. Use unscented laundry and personal care products. Perfumed menstrual pads, laundry detergent, fabric softener, even scented dryer sheets could inflame the genital area and cause itching or burning. Most products have an unscented version. For instance, Dreft detergent is made for babies and those with ultra-sensitive skin. You can also find unscented Purex laundry detergent, Downy fabric softener, dryer sheets, etc. Even store brands often have an unscented version of these products.

17. Douche with caution. While douching under a doctor's care can be helpful for certain conditions, be careful when self-treating. Douching can create a pH imbalance in your vagina. Good as well as bad bacteria are washed out. Follow your doctor's instructions for douching. Always use an unscented douche.

18. Wash your vulvar/vaginal area with water only. Strange as that might sound, the vagina and vulva don't need more than that. Soap can upset the balance of vaginal flora and increase symptoms.

19. Use unscented soap (such as pure oatmeal) if you feel water isn't enough. For some women, these products cleanse without causing irritation. But please read

the label to be sure there are no additional ingredients to which you are sensitive. For instance, some women have found glycerin, a common ingredient in unscented soaps, to be drying and cause flare-ups.

20. Bend over when rinsing your hair in the shower so shampoo will not run down over your vulvar area. Chemical ingredients and scented products can cause a reaction when coming in contact with your genitals.

21. Wipe the rectal area properly. Vaginal infections can be caused by bacteria from the rectum. Wipe from front to back. This is another reason to change your underwear often. Bacteria may remain on underwear after a bowel movement.

22. Beware of routine genital shaving. Shaving too close to the vaginal lips can be chronically irritating and is not recommended. "Trimming" longer hair in that delicate area may be all you need for comfort and appearance.

Topical Remedies

23. Consider vaginal vitamin E suppositories to soothe inflammation. Before using, check the label to see if you have any known sensitivity to the ingredients. Many brands are made from soy or palm oils.

24. Apply prescription strength 5% Lidocaine ointment just at the vaginal opening once a day. All you need is a small dab on your fingertip, which you apply while gently opening your labial lips with your other hand. Be prepared—if you are in the right spot it may burn like crazy for one to two minutes when you first put it on, especially if you are having a flare-up. The good news is that as you heal, this reaction will lessen or disappear entirely. You'll need a doctor's prescription to get this product. Please do not substitute with seemingly similar off-the shelf products. They are just not the same. Most have additional irritating ingredients. You may want to have your doctor or nurse practitioner show you with a mirror exactly where to apply the Lidocaine. A picture or explanation is often not sufficient. Lidocaine ointment (5%) has been shown in controlled studies (such as one conducted by the Department of Obstetrics and Gynecology at the University of North Carolina School of Medicine) to be highly effective in reducing painful sexual penetration (dyspareunia). While there is immediate relief for some women, it can take up to six weeks or more of regular use for others to feel the positive effects. Lidocaine will not adversely affect your sexual partner. NOTE: Some experts are now prescribing a cream that combines two antinerve pain medications and a muscle relaxant, which has the advantage of soothing without burning.

Supplements

25. Think about taking calcium citrate. This form of calcium is thought to reduce acidity in the body. Calcium citrate is generally used in conjunction with a low acid or low oxalate diet, both of which are explained in the Diet section of this booklet.

26. Consider using Prelief. This over-the-counter product is made by the creators of Lactaid and Beano. It safely neutralizes the acidity of both foods and drinks. Acidity appears to be one major factor in escalating the sexual pain syndrome. While women with sexual pain are encouraged to follow a low-acid diet, it's not always possible. Prelief seems to be effective for many women when taken with meals, coffee, or other food and beverages.

27. Add fiber to your diet to promote regular bowel movements. Irritable bowel syndrome (IBS) can contribute to sexual pain when constipation is involved because of the pressure and added nerve sensitivity to the bladder and sexual organs. Reducing this pressure and sensitivity may provide some relief for painful sexual symptoms. Natural fiber comes from eating such foods as whole grains, fruits, vegetables, nuts, and seeds. Additional options for supplemental fiber are psyllium, flax, and a palatable over-the-counter product called Benefiber. However, some women may be sensitive to these products. Single ingredient cellulose powder, such as that made by NutriCology, Inc. may be your best option. Start with a very small amount and work your way up to the recommended usage. You may need to experiment until you find what works best for you.

28. Ensure bowel regularity. Magnesium oxide (a mineral) has been reported to be a gentle laxative. Those made by Nature Made have few extra ingredients in them. Miralax is another mild laxative product that is now sold over the counter as well.

29. Use caution with supplements. Look at the ingredient list of all vitamins and herbs before buying. For example, vitamin C, a common ingredient in supplements, is very acidic and known to cause symptom flare-ups.

Diet

30. Avoid caffeine. Many caffeinated products such as coffee, tea, and soda are also highly acidic and can be extremely irritating to bladder and genital tissues. Therefore, they are among the most agreed-upon substances for women with sexual pain to avoid.

31. Use caution, even with decaffeinated coffee, tea, and soda. It's not so much the caffeine as the acids in these products. Even a small amount of acid (such as in decaffeinated products) may adversely affect your symptoms. There are a number of coffee and tea brands claiming to be 90–100% acid-neutralized, such as Kava and Euromild coffees, and most herbal teas. Many teas touted for their health benefits, such as bancha, kukicha, green, and white tea, contain caffeine.

32. Be aware that medications may be high in acid content. For instance, aspirin and ibuprofen are high in acidity, and even though they may be enteric-coated to protect your stomach lining, the acids are still excreted through your kidneys and into your urine very quickly. If you need to take such medications, just be aware that they may worsen your pelvic and sexual discomfort.

33. Realize that chocolate contains acid, too. While it may be your favorite food in the world, eating those scrumptious treats might not be worth the resulting discomfort.

34. Understand that carbonated water or caffeine-free soda can also wreak havoc. Even with ice to dilute it, some people react negatively to plain old carbonated water. Soda, whether artificially sweetened or not, is too acidic for most women who suffer with conditions such as interstitial cystitis. Carbonated water can trigger not only the burning, but also irritable bowel and urinary urgency.

35. Beware of cranberry and other high-acid juices. Drinks like cranberry and orange juice are highly concentrated acidic products. Even though many women with urinary tract infections do find relief with cranberry juice, IC sufferers have an entirely different condition though symptoms may feel the same.

36. Get rid of artificial sweeteners. These chemical alternatives can cause more health problems than you might imagine. For sexual pain sufferers, the issue that matters here is the potential irritation to your bladder and vaginal/vulvar area.

37. Minimize the use of alcoholic drinks. Some products, such as red wines, cordials, and mixed drinks with soda, fresh lemon, or lime, are particularly acidic and irritating.

38. Drink a lot of water. Remember that plain old water can be your best friend. It's one of the kindest things you can do for your body overall. Acidic urine can irritate already inflamed and tender vulvar/vaginal tissues. Water further dilutes the acid concentration in your urine and can relieve burning and pain during sexual activity. Water helps relieve constipation, joint pains, headaches, interstitial cystitis, and much more. Drink bottled or filtered water rather than tap water because additional chemicals may be added to regular drinking water.

39. Test out a low-acid diet. Based on the theory that acidity increases the burning of urine and causes other conditions to flare up (such as irritable bowel, interstitial cystitis, and vaginal/vulvar pain), women with sexual pain are strongly encouraged to try the low-acid diet. Here are a few suggestions for the Low-Acid Diet.

Generally OK
Broccoli, Cottage cheese, Cream cheese, All fresh meat, fish, eggs, turkey, etc., Millet, Oatmeal, All cooking oils, Parsley, Pears, Rice, Snow peas, Spring water, Squash

Possibly OK
Almonds, Apple juice, Avocado, Bananas, Buttermilk, Honeydew, Onion, Parmesan cheese, Rye bread, Spinach, Sunflower seeds

Avoid
Apricots, Aged cheese, Citrus fruits and drinks, Grapes, Cured meats (unless preservative-free—usually found in the health food store), Most nuts, Soybeans, Soy milk, Wine, Yogurt

40. Explore a low-oxalate diet for vulvodynia and vestibulitis. Oxalates are known to cause kidney stones. There is a theory that oxalates also cause/contribute to sexual pain conditions such as vulvodynia. There are many women who have found this food plan helpful. However, there is conflicting evidence and no proven correlation between oxalates in one's food/body and sexual pain flare-ups, except anecdotally. Here are a few suggestions for a low-oxalate diet:

Generally OK
Avocado, Berries, Cauliflower, Meat, poultry, fish, eggs, Melons, Milk, low-fat Mushrooms, Nectarines, Oatmeal, Rice

Possibly OK
Apple, Apricots, Asparagus, Broccoli, Carrots, Cherries, Cornbread, Parsnips, Pears, Pineapple

Avoid
Beer, Black/blueberries, Celery, Green beans, Green peppers, Grits, Most nuts, Parsley, Peanut Butter, Potatoes, sweet Raspberries, Rhubarb, Strawberries, Tangerines, Tofu

41. Determine your own food triggers by using a food/pain diary chart. There are some differences between the low-acid and low-oxalate food lists. If you have multiple conditions that contribute to sexual pain, it may seem daunting to discover what your personal triggers are. Writing down what you eat and how your body reacts will make the detective work far easier. (We have developed a pain trigger diary that may help you. For more information, go to www.secretsuffering.com.)

42. Finding foods that bother you is a process of elimination. Everyone's chemistry is different. Some foods on the acceptable list may throw you into a flare-up within hours and some "avoid" foods may not bother you at all. Unlisted foods may also aggravate symptoms (such as certain spices). You are the best judge of which foods cause you a problem.

43. Eliminate entirely those foods that most bother you for a few weeks or longer. After you feel better, you can slowly begin incorporating the foods that you love into your diet. You will learn your threshold of discomfort. Some women find that eating a small amount of bothersome food infrequently may cause little or no symptoms. It becomes a balancing act. You know your own pain tolerance. Back off when you've reached it.

44. Be diligent and conscientious about following these diet suggestions for a while. While it's possible that you will find no correlation between food/drinks and your symptoms, it's well worth the time and effort to see if this simple change in your eating makes an impact on your chronic sexual pain syndrome.

45. Remember that locating trigger foods is not a quick fix. You've suffered far too long, but it's still going to take some time to figure out your personal triggers, if any.

46. Keep your diet simple and healthy. Eat foods with the least number of ingredients, like steamed vegetables, whole fruit, and grilled fish. Doing so will also make it easier to avoid triggers.

47. Read ingredient labels. Some of the biggest offenders are foods that are hidden in the ingredient list. Wheat is one of the more prevalent and bothersome ingredients for women with chronic sexual pain. Flour products, whole-grain or not, are in a vast number of foods besides bread, pancakes, and pasta. Unexpected examples of products containing wheat are soy sauce, some cheeses, gravy, and veggie burgers.

48. Vary your food choices to help determine food triggers. Eat different foods from meal to meal and day to day. Isolate foods as much as possible to learn which cause the most problems. Better yet, rotate your foods to strengthen your overall health. This ensures you maintain adequate amounts of vitamins and minerals and provides the nutrition you need.

Traditional Medical Treatments

49. Consider a medical approach. It can take a combination of treatments to significantly relieve sexual pain. Hopefully, more and more doctors will become experts in diagnosing and treating sexual/pelvic pain syndrome and integrate with other types of health care providers to provide a complete approach for recovery from this debilitating condition.

50. Use surgery cautiously for the conditions described in this Appendix. Learn as much as possible about your symptoms, their causes, and what might help. Be your best advocate for care.

51. Educate your doctor. Aid your health care provider in understanding how to treat your condition as you learn more about what triggers your sexual pain. The professional is there to help and may be glad to receive new information. Relieving nonspecific sexual/pelvic pain can be a stubborn, challenging, frustrating road, even for the best of doctors and patients. Sometimes doctors run out of ideas. A good doctor will be happy to learn about additional alternatives and refer you to an appropriate specialist if necessary.

52. Research estrogen. Some peri- and postmenopausal women have found relief from vaginal pain during intercourse by using estrogen vaginal supplements. For example, the Estring is a device that a woman inserts into her vagina that excretes small amounts of estrogen to enhance vaginal health (thereby decreasing dryness). Other women simply insert a small amount of estradiol cream or a slow release tablet, such as Vagifem (containing plant-derived estrogen), inside the vagina per their doctor's dosage recommendation. In addition, a compounding pharmacist can create customized formulations that do not contain ingredients to which you react. Note: As with the use of any hormones, consider carefully the risks prior to using them. Always use hormonal treatments under the care of a qualified health care practitioner.

53. Explore tri-cyclic antidepressants. Small doses of tri-cyclic antidepressants such as Amytriptyline (Elavil) and Nortriptyline (Pamelor) have worked to dull the vaginal and vulvar nerves. This can help reduce or even eliminate sexual pain, depending on the cause.

54. Be aware that some antiseizure medications have been shown to reduce sexual pain. Gabapentin (Neurontin) and Pregabalin (Lyrica) are two antiseizure medications commonly used by pain management practitioners to decrease other types of nerve-generated pain such as that which occurs with migraine, fibromyalgia, and myofascial spasm. These same medications can be carefully and safely utilized for pelvic and sexual pain if your doctor is familiar with their use.

55. Investigate Elmiron, a medication that helps reduce bladder inflammation and consequently lowers the pain of sexual penetration associated with interstitial cystitis. Elmiron is believed to help repair and restore the damaged bladder lining. While it can take a few months to notice the difference, women who have found success with this medication describe its effect as miraculous.

56. Notice medication side-effects related to sexual pain. Some medications, such as certain decongestants, may cause or increase bladder-triggered vaginal pain. Discuss your symptoms with your doctor, who may find an alternative if your sexual pain is worsened by specific medication.

57. Find a good sex therapist who understands chronic pelvic pain syndrome. This person can greatly assist you and your partner as a couple in regaining or maintaining intimacy despite the challenges.

58. Be aware that this type of sex therapy is a form of counseling focusing on actions and resolving psychological issues, leading couples to increased intimacy. Among these issues is fear of pain. Both may be afraid to initiate sex. The partner may be fearful of causing pain and the patient apprehensive and closed off in anticipation of pain. Note: There are also psychologists and other types of therapists who specialize in sexual pain issues.

Stress Relief

59. Consider meditation. It can make a big difference. Stress relief is an important component in treating sexual pain. Meditation can be an easy, simple way to experience relaxation and help you learn to cope with your discomfort.

60. Learn to relax through pelvic floor biofeedback. Biofeedback treatment for pelvic floor dysfunction utilizes machinery hooked up to your body that helps train you to relax tight muscles. More and more physical therapists are incorporating this type of treatment into their practice for patients with sexual pain.

Intimacy

61. Schedule a weekly date with your partner. Even if you're having difficulties around sex, maintaining emotional intimacy with your partner will help relieve the tension. Setting aside a few hours a week to snuggle, watch movies, or share an adventure will keep you connected. Alternate with your partner to select activities you can both enjoy. Sex is not the only way to have fun and stay close.

62. Experiment. There are many exciting and fun ways to have sex even if you are unable to have intercourse. Sometimes men, and even women, feel that intercourse is the only "real" way to have sex and experience intimacy. Open your mind and that of your partner to sharing other types of sexual activity.

63. Understand that many women have lost interest in sex, often due to the pain they experience. Chances are you will relax and eventually enjoy sex again if you are willing to engage in sexual activity with your partner that does not cause you pain.

64. Realize that intimacy is a result of two people working together to please each other. While some men may say that only intercourse is "real" sex, many also admit that they get aroused by making their partner excited, with or without intercourse.

Appendix B

PELVIC PAIN AND URGENCY/FREQUENCY PATIENT SYMPTOM SCALE (PUF) AND VULVAR PAIN QUESTIONNAIRES

The following two questionnaires will put you in touch with very specific aspects of your pain and give you tremendous insight as to how your pain impacts your life. These are not tools for self-diagnosis, but important instruments to help you educate and work with your doctor on your specific elements of pelvic pain.

USING THE PUF SCALE TO DETECT SYMPTOMS OF IC*

After years of research into bladder pain, Dr. C. Lowell Parsons developed the PUF scale, a simple eight-question screening tool. By studying patients, he discovered that the presence of potassium penetrating the lining of the bladder caused symptoms such as urinary frequency and burning when no infection was present. According to Dr. Parsons, "If you have a bad mucous lining, you suck up potassium into the bladder wall, and you get symptoms."[1]

Prior to the creation of the PUF scale, the standard diagnostic procedure for IC was a potassium sensitivity test (PST), which involved injecting potassium directly into the bladder, sometimes a highly painful procedure. The questionnaire addresses pelvic pain (three questions), urinary urgency (two questions), urinary frequency (two questions), and sexual activity (one question). The answers to these questions help doctors determine if a patient is likely to test positive for potassium in their bladder without having to undergo the

---

*Pelvic and Urgency/Frequency Patient Symptom Scale © 2000 C. Lowell Parsons, MD. Reprinted with permission.

invasive test. Dr. Parsons made it clear that this is not an IC test, but a test that measures pelvic pain, frequency, and urgency. "However," he said, "overall, the majority of individuals who test high (10 or over) do have IC." In addition, Dr. Parsons conducted a study with gynecology (not urology) patients, showing that those who suffered with painful sex had a 92 percent chance of having a positive potassium test.[2]

Dr. Parsons said he wanted to keep the test simple: one page. It took over a year testing different iterations of the questionnaire before he was satisfied. For instance, he said, "We sat down with gynecologists and validated the questions against 334 patients."[3]

Following is the PUF scale. Take a moment to complete this questionnaire. Even if you think your pain has nothing to do with bladder symptoms, you may be surprised at the results.

Pelvic Pain and Urgency/Frequency Patient Symptom Scale

Please circle the answer that best describes how you feel for each question.

	0	1	2	3	4	Symptom Score	Bother Score
1 How many times do you go to the bathroom during the day?	3-6	7-10	11-14	15-19	20+		
2 a. How many times do you go to the bathroom at night?	0	1	2	3	4+		
b. If you get up at night to go to the bathroom, does it bother you?	Never Bothers	Occasionally	Usually	Always			
3 a. Do you now or have you ever had pain or symptoms during or after sexual intercourse?	Never	Occasionally	Usually	Always			
b. Has pain or urgency ever made you avoid sexual intercourse?	Never	Occasionally	Usually	Always			
4 Do you have pain associated with your bladder or in your pelvis (vagina, labia, lower abdomen, urethra, perineum, testes, or scrotum)?	Never	Occasionally	Usually	Always			

	0	**1**	**2**	**3**	**4**	**Symptom Score**	**Bother Score**
5 a. If you have pain, is it usually		Mild	Moder-ate	Severe			
b. Does your pain bother you?	Never	Occasionally	Usually	Always			
6 Do you still have urgency after going to the bathroom?	Never	Occasionally	Usually	Always			
7 a. If you have urgency, is it usually		Mild	Moder-ate	Severe			
b. Does your urgency bother you?	Never	Occasionally	Usually	Always			
8 Are you sexually active? Yes __ No __							
Symptom Score = (1, 2a, 3a, 4, 5a, 6, 7a)							
Bother Score = (2b, 3b, 5b, 7b)							
TOTAL SCORE (Symptom Score + Bother Score) =							

Total score ranges from 1 to 35.

A total score of 10–14 = 74% likelihood of positive a potassium sensitivity test (PST); 15–19 = 76%; 20 or above = 91% likelihood of a positive PST.

Combining symptoms with the degree to which they bother you, you come up with a score that can range from 1 to 35.

• A total score of 10–14 means that there is a 74% likelihood of a positive PST.
• A total score of 15–19 means that there is a 76% likelihood of a positive PST.
• A total score that is 20 or above represents a 91% likelihood of a positive PST.

A positive PST strongly indicates you have interstitial cystitis. However, you will want have a culture to rule out a kidney, bladder, or urinary tract infection. If there is no infection present and you still experience these symptoms, search for a doctor who knows how to diagnose and treat interstitial cystitis.

© 2000 C. Lowell Parsons, M.D. Reprinted with permission.

VULVAR PAIN QUESTIONNAIRE*

The following questionnaire was developed by three experts in the field of physical therapy: Kathie Hummel-Berry, PT, PhD; Kathie Wallace, PT; and Hollis Herman MS, PT, OCS.

Dr. Echenberg feels that this set of questions is extremely helpful in evaluating a number of issues that are interrelated regarding pelvic and sexual pain disorders. Again, it is not recommended for self-diagnosis, but as another excellent tool for your doctor to gather the necessary information to more specifically understand your symptom complexity. There is no need to score yourself, but obviously, the higher the score, the more extensive your problem could be.

Vulvar Pain Functional Questionnaire (V-Q)

These are statements about how your pelvic pain affects your everyday life. Please check one box for each item below, choosing the one that best describes your situation. Some of the statements deal with personal subjects. These statements are included because they will help your health care provider design the best treatment for you and measure your progress during treatment. Your responses will be kept completely confidential at all times.

1. Because of my pelvic pain
   - ❑ 3 I can't wear tight-fitting clothing like pantyhose that puts any pressure over my painful area.
   - ❑ 2 I can wear closer fitting clothing as long as it only puts a little bit of pressure over my painful area.
   - ❑ 1 I can wear whatever I like most of the time, but every now and then I feel pelvic pain caused by pressure from my clothing.
   - ❑ 0 I can wear whatever I like; I never have pelvic pain because of clothing.

2. My pelvic pain
   - ❑ 3 Gets worse when I walk, so I can only walk far enough to move around in my house, no further.
   - ❑ 2 Gets worse when I walk. I can walk a short distance outside the house, but it is very painful to walk far enough to get a full load of groceries in a grocery store.
   - ❑ 1 Gets a little worse when I walk. I can walk far enough to do my errands, like grocery shopping, but it would be very painful to walk longer distances for fun or exercise.
   - ❑ 0 My pain does not get worse with walking; I can walk as far as I want to
   - ❑ 0 I have a hard time walking because of another medical problem, but pelvic pain doesn't make it hard to walk.

3. My pelvic pain
   - ❑ 3 Gets worse when I sit, so it hurts too much to sit any longer than 30 minutes at a time.
   - ❑ 2 Gets worse when I sit. I can sit for longer than 30 minutes at a time, but it is so painful that it is difficult to do my job or sit long enough to watch a movie.
   - ❑ 1 Occasionally gets worse when I sit, but most of the time sitting is comfortable.
   - ❑ 0 My pain does not get worse with sitting, I can sit as long as I want to.
   - ❑ 0 I have trouble sitting for very long because of another medical problem, but pelvic pain doesn't make it hard to sit.

4. Because of pain pills I take for my pelvic pain

   ❑ 3 I am sleepy and I have trouble concentrating at work or while I do housework.

   ❑ 2 I can concentrate just enough to do my work, but I can't do more, like go out in the evenings.

   ❑ 1 I can do all of my work, and go out in the evening if I want, but I feel out of sorts.

   ❑ 0 I don't have any problems with the pills that I take for pelvic pain.

   ❑ 0 I don't take pain pills for my pelvic pain.

5. Because of my pelvic pain

   ❑ 3 I have very bad pain when I try to have a bowel movement, and it keeps hurting for at least 5 minutes after I am finished.

   ❑ 2 It hurts when I try to have a bowel movement, but the pain goes away when I am finished.

   ❑ 1 Most of the time it does not hurt when I have a bowel movement, but every now and then it does.

   ❑ 0 It never hurts from my pelvic pain when I have a bowel movement.

6. Because of my pelvic pain

   ❑ 3 I don't get together with my friends or go out to parties or events.

   ❑ 2 I only get together with my friends or go out to parties or events every now and then.

   ❑ 1 I usually will go out with friends or to events if I want to, but every now and then I don't because of the pain.

   ❑ 0 I get together with friends or go to events whenever I want, pelvic pain does not get in the way.

7. Because of my pelvic pain

   ❑ 3 I can't stand for the doctor to insert the speculum when I go to the gynecologist.

   ❑ 2 I can stand it when the doctor inserts the speculum if they are very careful, but most of the time it really hurts.

   ❑ 1 It usually doesn't hurt when the doctor inserts the speculum, but every now and then it does hurt.

   ❑ 0 It never hurts for the doctor to insert the speculum when I go to the gynecologist.

8. Because of my pelvic pain

   ❑ 3 I cannot use tampons at all, because they make my pain much worse.

   ❑ 2 I can only use tampons if I put them in very carefully.

   ❑ 1 It usually doesn't hurt to use tampons, but occasionally it does hurt.

   ❑ 0 It never hurts to use tampons.

   ❑ 0 This question doesn't apply to me, because I don't need to use tampons, or I wouldn't choose to use them whether they hurt or not.

9. Because of my pelvic pain

   ❑ 3 I can't let my partner put a finger or penis in my vagina during sex at all.

❑ 2 My partner can put a finger or penis in my vagina very carefully, but it still hurts.

❑ 1 It usually doesn't hurt if my partner puts a finger or penis in my vagina, but every now and then it does hurt.

❑ 0 It doesn't hurt to have my partner put a finger or penis in my vagina at all.

❑ 0 This question does not apply to me because I don't have a sexual partner.

❑ 0 Specifically, I won't get involved with a partner because I worry about pelvic pain during sex.

10. Because of my pelvic pain

❑ 3 It hurts too much for my partner to touch me sexually even if the touching doesn't go in my vagina.

❑ 2 My partner can touch me sexually outside the vagina if we are very careful.

❑ 1 It doesn't usually hurt for my partner to touch me sexually outside the vagina, but every now and then it does hurt.

❑ 0 It never hurts for my partner to touch me sexually outside the vagina.

❑ 0 This question does not apply to me because I don't have a sexual partner.

❑ 0 Specifically, I won't get involved with a partner because I worry about pelvic pain during sex.

11. Because of my pelvic pain

❑ 3 It is too painful to touch myself for sexual pleasure.

❑ 2 I can touch myself for sexual pleasure if I am very careful.

❑ 1 It usually doesn't hurt to touch myself for sexual pleasure, but every now and then it does hurt.

❑ 0 It never hurts to touch myself for sexual pleasure.

❑ 0 I don't touch myself for sexual pleasure, but that is by choice, not because of pelvic pain.

Appendix C

ABOUT THE INTERNET SURVEY CONDUCTED FOR *SECRET SUFFERING*

I began this project before meeting Dr. Echenberg by developing an online survey for women and their partners. I wanted to find out whether there was an even larger community experiencing my problems. After meeting the doctor and getting additional health care provider feedbacks, the survey that began with about 5 questions eventually grew to 32 questions for women and 12 for partners. Most were multiple choice with an option for additional comments. We kept the survey active from December 2006 through December 2007.

Because this is not a scientific survey, please take the results with a grain of salt. The survey software (PHPESP) was hosted on my site to further ensure privacy. The only identifier was the respondent's IP address, so I could remove duplicates. Further, there were some responses that were clearly spam, and I removed those as well.

Throughout *Secret Suffering*, you'll find a few comments from these anonymous survey respondents. I also used the survey as a way to recruit interviewees. Dr. Echenberg and I are very grateful to Christin Veasley, Associate Executive Director of the National Vulvodynia Association (NVA, http://www.nva.org), and to Howard I. Glazer, PhD (http://www.vulvodynia.com) for sending a request for participants through their newsletters, which garnered many respondents and willing interviewees.

From the final survey (data from previous iterations have a few hundred responses, which are not included), the total number of participants was approximately 700 patients and 80 partners (only one woman answered the partner survey). Again, bearing in mind that this survey was not scientific, here are a few statistics:

WOMEN'S SURVEY RESULTS

- 48 percent have experienced pain for over five years
- 32 percent (highest percentage) are between 21 and 30 years of age
- 41 percent consider the pain severe
- 74 percent describe one symptom as burning
- 58 percent says they have sex less than they used to
- 30 percent are less emotionally intimate
- 68 percent say intercourse hurts
- 51 percent say they continue with intercourse even when it hurts
- 71 percent say these conditions make them feel depressed/despondent
- 41 percent have seen five or more health care providers
- 63 percent were overall unsatisfied with the care they received from health care providers

PARTNER'S SURVEY RESULTS

- 73 percent say they feel badly for their partner
- 86 percent say their partner asks or tells them to stop if it hurts during sex
- 54 percent are disappointed
- 83 percent says this issue won't cause their relationship to end

You can download all the results and respondent's comments from the final survey in a PDF file at our Web site (http://www.secretsuffering.com/survey.pdf).

Appendix D

ABOUT THE EXPERTS INTERVIEWED FOR *SECRET SUFFERING*

In writing *Secret Suffering,* we wanted the input of leading researchers and practitioners in the field of chronic pelvic pain (CPP). We recruited these interviewees from the body of research in the field, the International Pelvic Pain Society (IPPS), e-mail correspondence with medical professionals who had heard about our work, and Dr. Echenberg's personal contact with such experts.

I interviewed a number of people in a variety of fields relating to sexual pain. The common thread between all the interviewees was a passion to help patients find relief from sexual pain and a willingness to go the distance to do so. Among these experts are some of the top professionals in pain research, interstitial cystitis (IC), pelvic pain, and related subspecialties.

It was truly an honor to speak to these giants in their field; however, I must admit that each time I picked up the phone to call one of these experts, I felt intimidated by the stature of these brilliant men and women and had a looming terror that I would sound like a complete fool. However, without exception, everyone with whom I spoke was warm, caring, good-natured, and completely without pretension. No matter how unschooled my questions, they answered patiently in language that I, as a layperson, could understand.

Overwhelmingly, these medical professionals were recruited or accidentally found themselves presented with pelvic and sexual pain patients and found a calling to help these suffering women (and men) unravel the mystery of this complex syndrome. In addition, I think it is no coincidence that each, whether researcher or practitioner, possessed the temperament, compassion, and patience required of those who are most effective in this field.

We have listed our experts in alphabetical order, with the exception of the late Dr. C. Paul Perry, who we honor first.

C. PAUL PERRY, MD, was medical director of the C. Paul Perry Pelvic Pain Center in Birmingham, Alabama. He was a practicing gynecologist for over 30 years and the founder of the IPPS. Dr. Perry was the author of dozens of scientific articles and has been cited in numerous medical journals and textbooks.

Dr. Perry was a man of tremendous religious faith. "About 12 years ago," he said, "I was led to drop my obstetrics practice and go into pelvic pain exclusively, and we've had a chronic pelvic pain clinic for about 10 or 12 years." This calling changed not only Dr. Perry's life, but also the lives of thousands of patients and medical professionals.

Dr. Perry was one of the most educated professionals in the field of CPP. His breadth of knowledge was vast, and he had a continued willingness to educate himself about the latest breakthroughs. Yet, he ended our interview by telling me, "My patients taught me 99 percent of everything I know."

Shortly after our interview, we found out that Dr. Perry had terminal cancer, and sadly, a few months later, he died. Dr. Perry was beloved by the patients he helped and the medical community he served through the IPPS. His service to disseminate his knowledge across the world will never be forgotten.

KAREN J. BERKLEY, PHD, is a neuroscientist and pelvic pain researcher. She is currently a McKenzie Professor in the program in neuroscience at Florida State University and is one of the preeminent researchers in the field of chronic pain, in which she focuses on endometriosis and the role of the central nervous system.

Dr. Berkley and her team have gained immense insight into how information feeds into the nervous system in a way that creates "cross-organ interaction within the context of the nervous system to create abnormal perceptions to stimulation of other organs in some individuals and not in others." Answers are crucial to understanding the connection between the nervous system and such chronic pain conditions as CPP, IC, endometriosis, irritable bowel syndrome, fibromyalgia, headache, temporomandibular disorder, and chronic fatigue syndrome and will lead to better and more effective treatment.

DANIEL BROOKOFF, MD, PHD, is the director of the Center for Medical Pain Management at Presbyterian–St. Luke's Medical Center in Denver, Colorado. He is certified by the American Board of Internal Medicine, with a subspecialty certification in medical oncology, and is a member of the American Pain Society.

Dr. Brookoff has been the principle investigator at site on over 20 commercially sponsored multisite research projects, several of which were investigator initiated, involving pharmaceutical and medical devices in pain and symptom management. He has also performed independent research on the endocrinologic effects of chronic pain and opioid analgesics. He has been called a hero in the field of IC and is widely published in the areas of pain management, drug complications, and pelvic pain.

SANDRA (SANDY) DIDONA, LPN, is a nurse who has worked in a variety of settings, including OB/GYN offices, nursing homes, a rehab hospital, hospice, and with surgical patients, pregnant women, and cancer patients during the course of her 20-year nursing career. She has worked with Dr. Echenberg in various capacities for over 15 years, caring for women as they experienced the joy of birth, the challenges of difficult diagnoses, and the sorrow of terrible loss.

The experiences they have had working together have created a bond that adds a quality of care that is a gift to the women who enter their chronic pelvic pain center. The biggest surprise for Sandy in working with women who suffer from chronic sexual and pelvic pain is that, "There are so many people out there who aren't being taken care of properly and find us at such a late stage. They're already over the fence, down the hill and run over by the car by the time they get to us. And then we have to do a lot of maintenance to get them back up the hill again."

LYNDSAY ELLIOTT, PHD, is a clinical psychologist with a pelvic pain specialty. Her office is located in Newport Beach, California. While doing both pre- and post-doctoral work at the University of California, Los Angeles, Dr. Elliott worked as a research associate in neurology and was a lecturer in pain management. She stays current on the latest research, and her professional memberships include the American Pain Society, International Association for the Study of Pain, American Academy of Pain Management, American Chronic Pain Association, and IPPS.

Dr. Elliott has found tremendous satisfaction in working with women who suffer from pelvic pain. As an expert in the field, she now receives referrals from a wide network of doctors. Though she has studied the field extensively, she said, "It's really through my patients that I learn the most."

LISA C. FOURNACE, MSN, APN, is a nurse practitioner at Heritage Women's Center in Nashville, She specializes in chronic pelvic pain and urogynecology.

When she was in school, the physician who was her preceptor had an interest in CPP, which rubbed off on her. After she graduated, she worked with him and grew more passionate about the field. She said, "I kept seeing more and more women who thought it was normal to have pain with intercourse or go to the bathroom every hour or to have a little bit of pain throughout the day. None of this is normal and women shouldn't have to accept it."

NEL GERIG, MD, is a urologist and IC specialist who practices in Denver, Colorado. Her passion for the field of CPP is partially due to the lack of doctors who will treat it. Luckily for many of her patients, those doctors in her area are willing to send them to her. When she first went into practice in 1998, Dr. Gerig was reticent about dealing with women's pelvic pain issues because there were few female urologists, and she said, "I didn't want to be pegged as 'the women's urologist.' I wanted to treat everyone. But women found me. Many of these women had interstitial cystitis and I felt ill-prepared to treat them."

Because she, as most doctors, was not educated in the complex treatment of CPP, Dr. Gerig dove head first into all available literature and training on the bladder aspect of pelvic pain, which is now called painful bladder syndrome/interstitial cystitis (PBS/IC).

LISA IACOVELLI, PT, is a physical therapist at her Physical Medicine Center of Marin in Mill Valley, California. She began her career in 1986 and came to her interest in the field of pelvic pain through her own experience. Initially, she treated primarily acute and chronic back and neck patients. However, she was personally having some issues with "irregular periods," which led to an increased interest in women's health.

She opened her physical therapy practice in the 1990s, and it was initially geared toward women suffering with pelvic pain, but she has been seeing more and more male patients. She is very grateful for the support of her own gynecologist and the other doctors who continue to refer patients to her. She said, "I had support because the doctors were interested in discovering what treatment was available because they were struggling with finding a way to treat these patients."

BRUCE KAHN, MD, FACOG, is a gynecologist with the Scripps Clinic Medical Group in San Diego, California. He is the director of Graduate Medical Education at Scripps Memorial Hospital, La Jolla, and an adjunct assistant clinical professor at the Uniformed Services University of the Health Sciences in Bethesda, MD. He coordinates clinical rotations at Scripps Hospitals for obstetrics and gynecology residents from the Naval Medical Center

San Diego, and together with his partners, he is preparing to launch a fellowship in minimally invasive gynecologic surgery in July 2009. He is a reviewer for the journals *Obstetrics & Gynecology, Hospital Physician,* and *Journal of Women's Health.*

Dr. Kahn has been involved in a number of studies on the relationship of interstitial cystitis and chronic pelvic pain. He lectures regionally and nationally on the diagnosis and treatment of chronic pelvic pain. He tries to take what is considered an extremely complicated topic and make it more easily understood by patients and practitioners alike. Dr. Kahn champions partnering with patients to develop treatment plans for pain management.

JUDY KURIANSKY, PHD, is an internationally renowned clinical psychologist and certified sex therapist, popular lecturer, newspaper columnist, and author. On the adjunct faculty of the Department of Counseling and Clinical Psychology, Columbia University Teachers College, and the Department of Psychiatry, Columbia College of Physicians and Surgeons at Columbia Medical Center, she was appointed visiting professor of Peking University Health Science Center in Beijing. She is also a representative to the United Nations for the International Association of Applied Psychology and the World Council for Psychotherapy, and she is on the executive board of the Committee on Mental Health.

Dr. Judy is the author of numerous relationship books, including *The Complete Idiots Guide to a Healthy Relationship* and *The Complete Idiots Guide to Tantric Sex.* Her most recent series is a four-volume set for Praeger Publishers on *Sexuality Education: Past, Present and Future.* The host of a popular call-in radio show for decades, she now gives wise advice to men and women of all ages at www.drjudy.com.

C. LOWELL PARSONS, MD, is professor of surgery at the University of California at San Diego and runs one of the largest IC clinics in the world. Dr. Parsons is a pioneer in the field of IC research and developed the Pelvic Pain and Urgency/Frequency Patient Symptom Scale, now often used as a standard diagnostic questionnaire for potential IC patients. In addition, he led the way to the discovery of Elmiron, which is a medication now used to repair the bladder lining in IC patients.

Dr. Parson's mission has been to put the pieces of the IC puzzle together to properly diagnose and treat patients with this debilitating condition. During his brilliant career, Dr. Parsons has seen over 7,000 patients and has published nearly 300 medical journal articles and book chapters.

JOHN F. STEEGE, MD, is a professor and chief of the Advanced Laparoscopy and Pelvic Pain division, Department of Obstetrics and Gynecology at the University of North Carolina at Chapel Hill. He has also held academic positions at Duke University Medical Center and Yale University School of Medicine. Dr. Steege's clinical interests include operative laparoscopy, including the development of new procedures such as laparoscopically assisted hysterectomy and protocols to prevent adhesion reformation following laparoscopic surgery. He is an expert in the diagnosis and treatment of CPP and has edited, authored, or contributed to over 60 journal articles, reviews, book chapters, and abstracts on pelvic pain as well as on such subjects as pelvic adhesions, laparoscopy, and the psychological aspects of gynecology.

Dr. Steege became interested in the field of CPP in the late 1970s. He joined the Duke faculty in 1977, and in addition to his OB/GYN residency, he participated in a one-year fellowship in human sexuality and trained in the Masters and Johnson's style of psychotherapy for sexual dysfunctions.

CHRISTIN (CHRIS) VEASLEY, is the associate executive director of the National Vulvodynia Association (NVA). In 1993, at the age of 18, Chris was diagnosed with vulvodynia. At that time, the NVA was just beginning to form. She reached out to get information for herself and started a support group in Wisconsin, where she served as support leader until she finished college.

From there, she moved to Baltimore to do research on vulvodynia at Johns Hopkins. At the same time, she became a member of the NVA's executive board and also ran the Washington, D.C., support group. Chris was a research assistant in the Department of Neurology at Johns Hopkins for three years, before she began her career with the NVA in 2000.

Appendix E

RUNNING A PELVIC
PAIN MANAGEMENT PROGRAM

Robert J. Echenberg, MD, FACOG

I believe that every community could have centers of excellence for the treatment of chronic pelvic pain (CPP) guided by a relatively small number of interested and easily trained experienced gynecologists. The last 10 to 15 years of professional life for clinicians who have already given up obstetrics could be exciting, challenging, lucrative, and extremely gratifying if they would learn and utilize the model of pelvic pain management presented throughout *Secret Suffering*.

Done correctly, these practices could thrive financially. With an exceptional specialized staff to assist with intake, ongoing management, and treatment, great numbers of women could be seen regularly to receive reimbursable, effective in-office procedures that are so vital to restoring their quality of life.

Although most of the conferences, texts, and professional publications exhort physicians and other health care professionals to work together in a multidisciplinary and multimodality fashion, it is quite rare to find such a center in one location for chronic pelvic pain. But that is the goal.

It is because of the complexities of tying many different approaches together into a coordinated program for CPP that there are so few centers throughout the United States that work as a single unit. There are even fewer privately run centers of this type outside of the larger academic institutions. Even these larger settings are few and far between because it is just too difficult to accomplish in a corporate-type setting. From my own personal experience and that of many others I have met along the way, the politics and funding of these types of centers are just not yet a priority—too many departments and too many budgets and cost centers to coordinate when there is a misperception that it is not profitable to do so.

A SMALL PRIVATE PRACTICE CAN THRIVE

In light of the difficulties inherent in creating a single center, our program has proven itself a workable solution within a private practice of one physician, three full-time employees, and two part-time employees, along with a growing network of specialists with whom we can work. The program is significantly profitable utilizing only routine compensation from private insurances and Medicare.

In our practice, we take a comprehensive look at the patient as a whole. We focus on the pelvic region from the umbilicus to the mid-thigh, including the bones, muscles, and nerves within the pelvis as well as the bowel, uterus, ovaries, and vulvar area. Our job is to closely investigate the functions of the nervous system and the daily or monthly functions of the pelvic organs.

Running a pain management center for the female pelvis requires a multidisciplinary, multimodality, and a multiorgan system approach. We work with specialized pelvic floor physical therapists, a nutritional counselor, psychological counselors, acupuncturist, and massage therapists and encourage our patients to utilize any relaxation or mind–body techniques that will tend to help their pain and tension (such as yoga and meditation).

We receive referrals from doctors within a wide geographic region for the diagnoses and management of interstitial cystitis, vulvodynia, vulvar vestibulodynia, pain of irritable bowel syndrome, failed treatments for pelvic endometriosis, and all types of sexual pain disorders.

I have developed a database of specialists in the various complementary fields who are like-minded about and open to collaborating on chronic pain patient care. There are more and more such practitioners. In fact, we have a multidisciplinary group that meets regularly for discussion and education. More and more of these groups are sprouting up throughout the country.

THE MULTIMODALITY TREATMENT APPROACH

The multimodality portion of the equation involves such treatments as physical therapy, pharmaceutical drugs for chronic pain such as antiseizure medications and some tri-cyclic antidepressants for the control of chronic neuropathic (nerve generated) pain, as well as the shorter term use of acute pain medications including nonsteroidal anti-inflammatory medications (NSAIDs), opioids as needed, and antihistaminic medications because of the inflammatory response to chronic pain. We also recommend various dietary changes in order to decrease the irritability of the bladder and bowel, as well as prescribing the use of specialized drugs such as pentosan polysulfate (Elmiron, which is used for the treatment of interstitial cystitis).

Also treating the triggers of pain in the pelvis requires the multiorgan system approach including the urinary bladder, lower bowel, and reproductive organs, along with the knowledge and skills to assess and treat the musculoskeletal and peripheral nerve issues that almost always accompany these chronic pain issues.

Since pain is the issue and pelvic pain has an association with a number of other systemic disorders such as fibromyalgia, temporomandibular joint (TMJ), myofascial trigger points and pain, and various autoimmune disorders such as Sjogren's Syndrome and lichen sclerosis, other specialists in such fields as rheumatology, dermatology, and neurology are helpful as well.

COMPONENTS OF A SUCCESSFUL CPP PRACTICE

In summary, following are the components that have made our practice successful and have enabled women to significantly enhance their quality of life.

- Spending extended time at the initial visit with those who suffer from this combination of symptoms—when complaints of pain are out of proportion to the physical findings—or when pain persists following other repeated medical or surgical therapies. The earlier we pick up on, or the earlier patients are referred in the course of their chronic illness, the quicker they respond and stay improved and can actually be discharged from the program. However, it is important to note that CPP providers will continue to care for a portion of patients with more severe and long-standing symptoms for a prolonged period of time.
- Utilizing detailed screening questionnaires involving location, intensity, timing, and triggering of the painful symptoms.
- Understanding how acute pain differs from chronic pain.
- Awareness of the current science within the field of chronic pain physiology:

  - That there is likely to be a genetic predisposition to chronic pain syndromes
  - That women more commonly have chronic pain syndromes than men
  - That estrogen enhances so-called neurogenic inflammation, which results in increased levels of pain from small amounts of stimuli (allodynia and hyperalgesia)
  - That there is a cumulative imprinting of pain neurochemistry in the central nervous system through a person's lifetime that can, under certain circumstances, turn into a chronic regional pain syndrome such as migraine, fibromyalgia, chronic fatigue, and chronic pelvic pain
  - That this cumulative imprinting can result from both physical and emotional trauma (surgical, accidental, or purposeful abuse)

- Recognizing that younger women with CPP often have a history of involvement with various sports such as gymnastics, dance, contact sports, track and field, etc.
- Knowledge that in CPP, any combination of dysfunctions of the bladder, gynecologic, or lower bowel can be visceral triggers that stimulate long-term irritative

neuropathic signals to the central nervous system in the lower lumbar and sacral regions and can then manifest as a chronic regional pain syndrome.

- Knowledge that myofascial spasm and pain are then secondary results of the central sensitization that leads to further enhancement of the chronic pain (pelvic floor dysfunctions and lower back, hip, and psoas pain disorders).
- Working knowledge of both acute and chronic pain pharmaceuticals (NSAIDs, short- and long-acting opioids, tri-cyclic antidepressants, anti-anxiety agents, and anticonvulsant medications).
- Utilization of as many office-based procedures and modalities as possible regarding pain management (bladder instillations, nerve blocks, trigger point therapies), rather than surgery as a first resort.
- Trained nurses to perform office-based procedures when appropriate, such as bladder instillations, which enables more patients to receive treatment without feeling rushed.
- Having a well-trained and empathetic staff to act as a team in helping to calm and care for these terribly stressed patients. This staff can conduct the lengthy intake interviews, which can expedite diagnoses prior to the patient being seen by the doctor.
- Developing a caring referral base that includes at least one urologist, gynecologist, gastroenterologist, orthopedist, neurosurgeon, general surgeon, colo-rectal surgeon, chiropractor, specialized pelvic floor physical therapists, rheumatologist, acupuncturist, deep myofascial therapist, psychologist, and psychiatrist.

FINAL THOUGHTS

I do believe that it is only a matter of time before third-party payers realize that chronic pain is costing our system far more than it should and that patients would benefit even more with the use of less expensive modalities and more quality time spent. The model of a chronic pelvic pain management center that we are currently operating is showing to be not only highly effective for these difficult patients, but it can be satisfactorily manageable for the clinician as well.

What we are showing now is that a combination of nonsurgical approaches, including good medical management, patient/doctor shared responsibility, multidisciplinary referrals, and the judicious use of office procedures such as bladder instillations for painful bladder syndrome, peripheral nerve blocks for pudendal and ilio-inguinal neuralgias, and trigger point therapies, all can be very effective, cost saving, and profitable.

I am frequently asked if we are studying and researching any of our findings. My answer to that is that in order to do proper studies in today's medical environment it is necessary to set up treatment protocols that generally study the effectiveness of one variable out of many. In fact, when patients do go to the larger and more prestigious academic institutions for their pelvic pain, many of them are placed on one specific protocol or another, rather than having an individualized treatment plan.

Further, this usually involves eliminating numbers of other variables for treatment and concentrating on only those under study. Also, comparison groups are usually needed for controls, so the patient often doesn't know if they are on the real thing or not (blinded studies).

Our chronic pelvic pain management center has been and remains a work in progress. There have been few models like it, and we have attempted to take the best parts of those of which we were aware. Our patients may well be the best judge of how well our program has been succeeding. Our statistics coming from intake and follow-up surveys reveal that we have very significantly impacted their pain and their quality of life. On average, even though we see a very difficult population of referred and otherwise failed pelvic pain patients, their average intake pain starts at 8 out of 10 and falls later to an average of 3 out of 10. Their quality of life, on average, correspondingly rises from 3 out of 10 to 8 out of 10. So it is no wonder that I have fallen in love with my work all over again. It is our greatest hope that doctors will take notice of the urgent need, opportunity, and potential for professional and personal fulfillment that specialization in the care of CPP patients brings.

Appendix F

AN INTERNATIONAL PLEA

Recently, we received an e-mail from the creators of the first Web site on vulvodynia and pelvic pain in Poland. They wrote:

> In the work of creating our site, we found your website. We have also been reading your posts at the http://www.secretsuffering website and found your experience in helping women with chronic pelvic pain very impressive. We would like to ask you whether you could support our project here in Poland by giving us an interview about vulvodynia and other chronic pelvic pain conditions, which we would then translate into Polish and present to our readers on our site?
>
> Agnieszka Serafin and Mikolaj Czyz (psychologists)

In October 2008, Dr. Echenberg gave that interview. The following response from Agnieszka Serafin indicates the universality of the pelvic and sexual pain problems that are described throughout our book. Many of the challenges that they face abroad (in this case, Eastern Europe) are very similar to those we face here in America even today.

> Dear Dr. Echenberg,
> Thank you once again for the interview—we were both very impressed with it. After our talk, I felt that I would like to share with you a bit about our idea of working with women who suffer from vulvodynia and other types of chronic pelvic and sexual pain.
> We are the authors of the first website about vulvodynia in Polish. We are both psychotherapists and have an educational background in psychology, sociology, and management. Among other things, would like to focus on working with women

who suffer from vulvodynia and sexual pain. There is very little medical help and psychological support for such women in Poland.

Their situation is usually extremely difficult and lonely. Although we have been searching, we haven't yet managed to find a Polish doctor who diagnoses and treats vulvodynia. Women who write to us have usually been suffering from chronic pelvic pain for many years and are desperately trying to find help.

I am a psychologist and I really love my work; it fascinates me and surprises me all the time. But as much as I believe in the power of our psyche, emotions, dreams, and so on, I also know for sure that some things cannot be viewed just on the individual and psychological level. It would make no sense for us to try to offer only psychological help for this group of women, because what is desperately needed right now in Poland is raising public and medical awareness of female sexuality in general and chronic pelvic pain in particular.

I value psychotherapy greatly, but I am sure that it alone isn't enough to deal with chronic pelvic pain, because what is also really needed is the acknowledgment of doctors here and their willingness to try to help this group of women.

Unfortunately, when asked about the term "vulvodynia," the doctors that we have contacted here so far usually reply either that they don't know about it or that it is a psychological word used for pain that has no physical reason (and so there is no point for the medical world to take interest in it).

That is why we have created a website that not only contains a lot of information about the psychological aspects of vulvodynia and sexual difficulties, but also many medical pages (that I wrote myself, based on English and Scandinavian literature, but with some help from my mother, who is a doctor). We have sent information about the website to hundreds of doctors here, the media, physiotherapists, and so forth, but the response has been very scarce, which is, of course, frustrating to us, but we also understand that this is going to be a long process.

What is good is that the website has been on-line for a few months and we now have about a hundred visitors a day. In addition, many Polish women write about their experiences on the forum that we have created as part of the website. That's quite amazing for a sickness that nobody here knows exists! :)

I really believe that acknowledgment and validation of the pain is one of the most important aspects of any kind of healing, and I am very happy that the website is beginning to be such a place for some women who suffer. At the same time, the desperation and pain that they write about (years and years of lonely pain with no help from the medical world, lost jobs, ruined relationships and marriages, and so forth) really make us believe that the only way of addressing this problem effectively is by combining medical, social, and psychological help and support. Talking to you and realizing that it is possible for a doctor and a psychologist to have similar attitudes and priorities was such a wonderful experience to us!

Our hope is that in the future a place will be created here where Polish women will be able to get proper, multidisciplinary help; where there would be doctors, who would like to help them and listen to them, and who will work in tandem with physiotherapists and psychotherapists; a place that would give hope, but would also seek the cooperation and involvement of the women themselves, so that they could take an active part in their treatment and search for healing, and not only be passive "objects" to be treated.

I really believe in the power of getting involved in one's own healing—I know by now that it doesn't always mean you will get completely cured, but what it means to me is that you don't leave yourself in the pain, you try to be there for yourself and find the support, comfort, and inner power that you so long for when you are sick. This is, of course, nearly impossible to do when nobody believes in your pain. Therefore, what is needed right now is to focus on the social aspect, media etc.

We realize that such a dream will be very, very difficult to fulfill for many reasons—lack of interested professionals, lack of finances, lack of experience in this field, the paradigm in which the most important thing is to quickly get as many patients consulted as possible (which means that there is no time to talk to the patients). But at the same time, I believe in the power of dreams.

One day—when there will also be others engaged in the social aspect of this work—I myself would love to focus on the psychological aspects of chronic female pain and sexuality. We would also like to create support groups for these women and work with couples, because any chronic pain, and this type in particular, of course, makes it very, very tough for a relationship to survive and maintain intimacy. Both Mikolaj Czyz and I are certified to work with individuals, couples, and groups, and we work under the supervision of Polish and American supervisors, licensed teachers of Process Oriented Psychology.

In the end, I hope and believe that for a woman, the process of dealing with this type of sickness can not only be a chance to treat the physical pain, but also for her to discover on this journey what is truly important to her in her womanhood, dreams, sexuality and values in life.

That's why I am so excited about this work and I hope I will get the chance to explore it further with many women.

With kind regards,
Agnieszka Serafin

URL: (In Polish) http://www.vulvodynia.pl

(Translated to English)
http://translate.google.com/translate?u=http%3A%2F%2Fwww.vulvodynia.pl&sl=pl&tl=en&hl=en&ie=UTF-8

GLOSSARY

Acute pain: Pain that occurs as a direct result of tissue injury. Acute pain is an essential protective warning mechanism for alerting an individual to such injury and as a protective mechanism from further injury or death.

Adhesion: Scarring or sticking of structures together (adhering) because of previous inflammation or surgery.

Alcock's Canal: Tiny ligamental tunnel through which the pudendal nerve travels just before fanning out into the vulvar region. There is one on each side of the pelvis.

Biopsychosocial: Viewing biological, psychological, and social factors as all playing a significant role in human functioning in the context of disease or illness.

Bladder instillation: A treatment for interstitial cystitis to soothe the bladder. The doctor inserts a small amount of medication into the bladder through a tiny catheter. There are different formulations of medication utilized by doctors.

Bladder lining dysfunction: *See* Interstitial cystitis (IC).

Cauterization of endometriosis implants: Electrical or lasering of implants (the endometrial cells that attach themselves outside the uterus) on the surfaces of the abdominal and pelvic structures, usually done for the treatment of pain or infertility.

Central nervous system: Brain and spinal cord.

Chronic pain: Pain that is present over time (more than three months) and can be constant or intermittent. Chronic pain may vary in intensity, duration, and frequency and serves no physiologic protection to the individual, i.e., pain may be present long after tissue injury is healed.

Chronic pelvic pain (CPP): A regional pain syndrome involving noncyclic pain in the pelvis (all structures between mid-abdomen to mid-thigh, such as muscles, nerves and organs), characterized by combinations of dysfunctions of urologic, gynecologic, gastrointestinal, myofascial, and neuropathic (pain or discomfort generated from nerve injury or dysfunction) components.

Clitoris: Vulvar structure that responds with sexual pleasure upon physical stimulation. It can be highly sensitive and even painful in some women with chronic pelvic pain.

Culture: Collection of bodily fluid or tissue such as vaginal discharge or urine in order to test it for bacterial, viral, or fungal infections.

Cystoscopy: Scope inserted into the urethra and bladder for either testing bladder function or searching for pathology, such as cancer, inflammation, polyps, or urinary stones.

Dilator: Instruments to help stretch or dilate particular bodily passageways, such as the vagina or urethra. Vaginal dilators can be particularly helpful for women with pelvic floor dysfunction and sexual penetration pain when their physician or physical therapist instructs them properly on how to do so.

Dyspareunia: Pain or discomfort upon sexual penetration of the vagina.

Endometriosis: Common medical condition in women that is characterized by growth beyond or outside the uterus of tissue resembling endometrium, the tissue that normally lines the uterus; it may be associated with cyclic pelvic pain and is a common finding in women with infertility.

Fascia: Soft tissue component of the connective tissue throughout the body, providing strength and stability to the attachments between muscles and bone.

Fibromyalgia: A chronic disorder characterized by widespread pain, tenderness, and stiffness of muscles. Typically accompanied by fatigue, headache, and sleep disturbances. Trigger points (specific spots tender to touch) in muscle tissue are often thought to be associated with fibromyalgia and can activate pain.

High tone pelvic floor myofascial pain: *See* Pelvic floor hypertonic dysfunction.

Honeymoon cystitis: Outdated concept that assumed bacterial infections of the bladder were common with frequent sexual relations. Infections following sex are actually very uncommon. Symptoms of bladder irritation following sexual activity are more commonly due to flares of interstitial cystitis.

Hysterectomy: Surgical removal of the uterus (independent from removal of ovaries). Procedure may be done through the abdomen, vagina, or through laparoscope. Sometimes the cervix, which is part of the uterus, is not removed with a hysterectomy.

Imprinted pain: Cumulative long-term laying down of neurochemical memories within the nervous system following all types of painful injuries in our lives (physical and emotional, such as sports injuries or sexual abuse). These imprints can be reawakened by events in our lives and may contribute to various chronic pain syndromes.

Interferential (IF) unit: *See* Transcutaneous electrical nerve stimulator (TENS unit). The IF unit is a similar device used for pain, but with a different type of electrical current.

Interstitial cystitis (IC) (or painful bladder syndrome [PBS]: The presence of pain related to, and triggered by, a chronic inflammatory condition of the urinary bladder and accompanied by frequency and/or urgency. Nighttime awakening to urinate as well as sexual pain are also commonly associated symptoms.

Irritable bowel syndrome (IBS): Chronic functional disorder of the colon that is of unknown cause. IBS is characterized by diarrhea or constipation, or diarrhea alternating with constipation, abdominal pain or discomfort, abdominal bloating, and passage of mucus in the stool.

IVP (intravenous pyelogram): Specialized x-ray of kidneys looking for kidney abnormalities. Kidney ultrasound is used much more commonly today.

Kegel exercises: Tightening and releasing of pelvic floor muscles. This exercise is similar to stopping the flow of urine. Kegel exercises are commonly used after vaginal childbirth to help strengthen the pelvic floor. They are also used for individuals with stress urinary incontinence to avoid leakage. These exercises may not be appropriate when the muscles are already in pain and in spasm, as in hypertonic pelvic floor dysfunction, and should be used with caution and optimally under the proper supervision of specialized pelvic floor physical therapists.

Labia: External lips of the vulva. There are outer major lips, and inner minor lips.

Laparoscopy: Procedure that allows surgeons to view and surgically operate on the inside of the abdominal and pelvic cavities without making any major incisions (also called *minimally invasive surgery*).

Lesions: Generalized term that refers to any abnormal visual or palpable growth, scar, or marking anywhere in the body.

Lichen sclerosis: A common skin condition (dermatosis) that affects the external female genitalia, and less commonly elsewhere in the body, now considered an autoimmune disorder that slowly causes increasingly severe inflammation in the tissue. Scarring and adhesions around the labial lips and clitoris often occur over the years with a loss of the normal anatomic appearance of the vulva. Symptoms may range from none to very severe itching and even pain from the damage to the skin surface. It does not extend into the vagina. Lichen sclerosis is felt to be found more frequently in women with chronic pelvic pain and may well be yet another long-term irritant that leads to nerve sensitization. This condition is commonly under-diagnosed and under-treated.

Mittelschmerz: Pain or discomfort associated with mid-cycle ovulation.

Myofascial massage: Specialized therapeutic massage working on trigger points, designed to release spasmed muscles and fascia.

Neurochemical: Refers to chemicals within the nervous system that facilitate the transmission or inhibition of signals within us that control virtually all of our bodily functions and sensation.

Neurochemical memory: *See* Imprinted pain. This phenomenon is also felt to cause more and more sensitization within the nervous system that eventually works against us and may cause all types of chronic pain to become even more intense (e.g., migraine, fibromyalgia, CPP, and TMJ).

Neurogenic inflammation: A fairly new concept in the research world of chronic pain. Pain transmission through the nerves appears to cause an actual inflammatory response at those parts of the body to which those nerves are connected.

Neuropathic pain: Pain that is generating from the nervous system itself and not just because of acute tissue injury. Neuropathic pain is often a major component of chronic pain.

Nerve blocks: Any type of anesthetic block, such as that used prior to dental work, to prevent the sensation of pain. These types of blocks are called "peripheral" nerve blocks. Peripheral blocks used for CPP, such as pudendal and ilio-inguinal blocks, are not permanent but work to gradually desensitize nerve-generated pain when used in a series, over time. There are also central blocks, used more by back and pain management specialists. These are administered closer to the spinal cord.

Ovarian cyst: Any type of fluid-filled cavity on or within the ovary. Most cysts are common and are related to the normal ovarian hormonal cycle in preparation for the possibility of pregnancy every month. These cysts, related to ovulation, generally come and go on their own. Larger cysts that are persisting or are filled with complex solid and fluid components need to be investigated for more serious pathology. The vast amount of cysts do not cause any trouble at all and are *not* usually the cause of CPP.

Painful bladder syndrome (PBS): *See* Interstitial cystitis (IC).

Pelvic floor: All the muscles that surround and support the pelvic organs (uterus, bladder, and lower bowel).

Pelvic floor hypertonic dysfunction: Also called *high tone pelvic floor dysfunction.* Common syndrome of clenching and spasms of the pelvic floor and pelvic side wall muscles that results from, and ironically contributes significantly to, CPP.

Pelvic floor physical therapy: Specialized physical therapy for releasing the spasms and retraining of the pelvic floor, lower back, and contributing myofascial trigger points throughout the pelvic region. Both external and internal release techniques are used.

Pelvic organs: Urinary bladder, uterus, Fallopian tubes, ovaries, and lower bowel.

Perineum: The area of skin between the vaginal opening (in women), the base of the scrotum (in men), and the rectal opening.

Psoas muscle: Large muscles on either side of the spinal column, extending from the diaphragm down to the deep pelvis. These large muscles are very important in stabilizing and controlling all movements involved in our torso, such as pivoting, rotating, flexing, and extending on our pelvis and lower extremities. They can go into spasm and cause severe pain and are commonly overlooked, along with the pelvic floor core muscles, as major players in chronic recurrent and sometimes severe pelvic and sexual pain disorders. See Figure 2.2.

Pudendal block: This is a block injected into the pudendal nerve. *See* Nerve blocks.

Pudendal nerve: This nerve provides sensation to the entire vulva from the clitoris back to the anal opening. This nerve arises from the second, third, and fourth sacral nerves (nerves from the lower portion of your back, just above your butt), the same nerves that also connect to the sensory nerves from all of the pelvic organs. See Figures 4.1 and 4.2.

Pudendal neuralgia: Pain emanating from the pudendal nerve that may be a significant contributor to vulvodynia in some cases.

Regional pain syndrome: Chronic pain conditions that affect regions of the body, such as those that cause migraine, fibromyalgia, TMJ, and CPP. All regional pain syndromes share the fact that the central nervous system has become increasingly sensitized over time.

Sexual pain: Pain or discomfort resulting from any type of sexual activity. It is very important to realize that most sexual pain results from physical pain problems and is very uncommonly due to a mental or psychological disorder. Nonetheless, a great deal of anxiety, distress, depression, frustration, anger, and relationship issues can and often do arise secondarily from sexual pain disorders.

Somatic tissue: Muscles, nerves, ligaments, bone, connective tissues, and skin.

Temporomandibular joint disorder (TMJ): Acute or chronic inflammation and pain of the temporomandibular joint, which connects the lower jaw to the skull.

Transcutaneous electrical nerve stimulator (TENS unit): This device provides an electrical current through the skin for pain control. It essentially fools and diverts the brain's attention away from the focus of pain.

Trigger points: Tender, hyperirritable spots in the skeletal muscles (muscles that work with the skeletal system to facilitate motion) that are associated with nodules that can be felt in taut bands of muscle fibers. Trigger point researchers believe that palpable nodules are small contraction knots and a common cause of pain.

Trigger point therapies: Various techniques to release trigger points in muscle tissue to reduce the activation of pain.

Urinary tract infection (UTI): Infection and inflammation of the lower urinary tract (bladder and urethra) caused usually by bacterial organisms. Symptoms are often similar to those of interstitial cystitis, therefore, a urine culture should be done, whenever possible, to confirm whether there is a true infection prior to the onset of treatment.

Urethra: The tube leading from the bladder to the outside, through which urine is passed.

Urodynamics: Specialized studies of the bladder in order to distinguish between various functional bladder problems.

Vaginal infection: Common infections of the vagina, sometimes sexually transmitted, that can be easily diagnosed by a swab in the doctor's office and looked at under the microscope (bacterial vaginosis, yeast, trichomonas).

Vaginismus: Usually involuntary spasms of the pelvic floor muscles, sometimes resulting from residual emotional or psychological fears following previous physical or sexual abuse. This condition usually results in the inability to have any sort of vaginal penetration (such as intercourse, the use of tampons, or an internal gynecologic examination).

Vestibule: The vestibule is the vaginal opening, which contains large amounts of pain receptors.

Vestibulectomy: Surgical removal of the small strip of tissue between the vaginal lining and the outside skin of the vulva. The vestibule is the vaginal opening, which contains large amounts of pain receptors, and is the common location for neurogenic inflammation and pain with sexual penetration. Research is ongoing to help determine which women would most benefit from this type of surgical approach.

Visceral organs (pelvic): Urinary bladder, lower bowel, and reproductive organs.

Vulva: Area of the female anatomy that is bordered by the groin on either side, the rectal opening in the back, and the mons pubis and clitoris in the front.

Vulvar vestibulitis (vulvar vestibulodynia): Pain in the vestibule, usually at the back part of the vaginal opening that is now felt to be generated by highly sensitized nerve endings and contributed to by pelvic visceral triggers (conditions) such as IC, IBS, severe menstrual pain, stress, etc. This condition is frequently misdiagnosed and treated as a vaginal infection.

Vulvodynia: Chronic pain in the vulvar region. This can be broken down into vulvar vestibulodynia and generalized vulvodynia. The latter is less common and often very difficult to successfully treat. It is a deeper more generalized pain, can be spontaneous (unprovoked), or secondary to touch or pressure (provoked, such as by intercourse). The pain is variously described by patients as crawling, clenching, searing, painfully itching, stabbing, vice-like, hot-poker like, etc. Pain emanating from the pudendal nerve and its distribution may be a significant contributor to this condition in some cases (pudendal neuralgia).

NOTES

PREFACE

1. K. T. Zondervan, P. L. Yudkin, M. P. Vessey, M. G. Dawes, D. H. Barlow, and S. H. Kennedy, "Patterns of Diagnosis and Referral in Women Consulting for Chronic Pelvic Pain in UK Primary Care," *British Journal of Obstetrics and Gynaecology* 106 (1999): 1156–61.

CHAPTER 1

1. The names and many details of individuals discussed in this book have been changed to protect the patients' identities. Some of the stories are composites of patient interactions created for illustrative purposes. The biographies of our expert interviewees are contained in Appendix D.

CHAPTER 2

1. S. D. Mathias, M. Kuppermann, R. F. Liberman, R. C. Lipschutz, and J. F. Steege, "Chronic Pelvic Pain: Prevalence, Health-Related Quality of Life, and Economic Correlates," *Obstetrics and Gynecology* 87 (1996): 321–27.

2. International Association for the Study of Pain, "Global Year against Pain in Women—Real Women, Real Pain," http://www.iasp-pain.org/AM/Template.cfm?Section=Real_Women_Real_Pain&Template=/CM/HTMLDisplay.cfm&ContentID=4629; International Association for the Study of Pain, "Global Year against Pain in Women—Real Women, Real Pain: Fact Sheets," International Association for the Study of Pain, http://www.iasp-pain.org/AM/Template.cfm?Section=Fact_Sheets&Template=/CM/HTMLDisplay.cfm&ContentID=4448, esp. "Chronic Pelvic Pain Fact Sheet,"

http://www.iasp-pain.org/AM/Template.cfm?Section=Fact_Sheets&Template=/CM/ContentDisplay.cfm&ContentID=4506; Juan Diego Villegas-Echeverri and Claudia Camila Giraldo-Parra, "Chronic Pelvic Pain Associated with the Bladder: We Know It Exists but How Should We Name It?" *IPPS Newsletter* 15, no. 4 (2008), http://www.pelvicpain.org/news/pdfs/vol15_no4.pdf; see also the Web site of the International Pelvic Pain Society, http://www.pelvicpain.org.

3. M. K. Chung, R. P. Chung, and D. Gordon, "Interstitial Cystitis and Endometriosis in Patients with Chronic Pelvic Pain: The 'Evil Twins' Syndrome," *Journal of the Society of Laparoendoscopic Surgeons* 9, no. 1 (2005): 25–29.

4. C. L. Parsons, Jeffrey Dell, Edward J. Stanford, Michael Bullen, Bruce S. Kahn, Tracy Waxell, and James A. Koziol, "Increased Prevalence of Interstitial Cystitis: Previously Unrecognized Urologic and Gynecologic Cases Identified Using a New Symptom Questionnaire and Intravesical Potassium Sensitivity," *Urology* 60 (2002): 573–78.

5. C. L. Parsons and V. Tatsis, "Prevalence of Interstitial Cystitis in Young Women," *Urology* 64 (2004): 866–70; Parsons et al., "Increased Prevalence of Interstitial Cystitis."

6. Parsons and Tatsis, "Prevalence of Interstitial Cystitis."

7. Ibid.

8. Randy Pausch and Jeffrey Zaslow, *Last Lecture* (New York: Hyperion, 2008).

CHAPTER 4

1. K. J. Berkley, "A Life of Pelvic Pain," *Physiology and Behavior* 86 (2005): 272–80.

2. ACOG Practice Bulletin No. 51 with Fred Howard, "Chronic Pelvic Pain," *Obstetrics and Gynecology* 103 (2004): 589–605.

3. Fred M. Howard, C. Paul Perry, James E. Carter, Ahmed M. El-Minawi, and Rong-Zeng Lie, eds., *Pelvic Pain: Diagnosis and Management* (Philadelphia: Lippincott Williams and Wilkins, 2000), 55.

4. B. J. Collett, C. J. Cordle, E. R. Stewart, and C. Jagger, "A Comparative Study of Women with CPP, Chronic Nonpelvic Pain and Those with No Physical Pain Attending General Practitioners," *British Journal of Obstetrics and Gynecology* 105 (1998): 87–92.

CHAPTER 10

1. Michael Y. Sokolove, Warrior Girls—Protecting Our Daughters against the Injury Epidemic in Women's Sports (New York: Simon and Schuster, 2008).

2. Fred Howard, C. Paul Perry, James E. Carter, Ahmed M. El-Minawi, and Rong-Zeng Lie, eds., *Pelvic Pain: Diagnosis and Management* (Philadelphia: Lippincott Williams and Wilkins, 2000).

CHAPTER 12

1. A recommended book, David Wise and Rodney Anderson, *A Headache in the Pelvis—A New Understanding and Treatment for Prostatitis and Chronic Pelvic Pain Syndromes* (Occidental, CA: National Center for Pelvic Pain, 2008), points out that the prostate is blamed for many male pelvic pain patients. The authors have developed a program

primarily for the pelvic floor spasm and dysfunction, which is the most important aspect causing the pelvic pain itself. It has been successfully used with both men and women.

CHAPTER 13

1. Rachel P. Maines, The Technology of Orgasm: "Hysteria," the Vibrator, and Women's Sexual Satisfaction (Baltimore: The Johns Hopkins University Press, 1999).

2. C. L. Parsons, C. Greenspan, and S. G. Mulholland, "The Primary Antibacterial Defense Mechanism of the Bladder," *Investigations in Urology* 13 (1975): 72–78.

3. J. M. Teichman and C. L. Parsons, "Contemporary Clinical Presentation of Interstitial Cystitis," *Urology* 69 (2007): 41–47; C. L. Parsons, "The Role of the Urinary Epithelium in the Pathogenesis of Interstitial Cystitis/Prostatitis/Urethritis," *Urology* 69 (2007): S9–S16; C. L. Parsons, Jeffrey Dell, Edward J. Stanford, Michael Bullen, Bruce S. Kahn, and John J. Willems, "The Prevalence of Interstitial Cystitis in Gynecologic Patients with Pelvic Pain, as Detected by Intravesical Potassium Sensitivity," *American Journal of Obstetrics and Gynecology* 187 (2002): 1395–400.

4. ACOG Practice Bulletin No. 51 with Fred Howard, "Chronic Pelvic Pain," *Obstetrics and Gynecology* 103 (2004): 589–605.

APPENDIX B

1. C. L. Parsons, Paul C. Stein, Mohamed Bidair, and Diana Lebow, "Abnormal Sensitivity to Intravesical Potassium in Interstitial Cystitis and Radiation Cystitis," *Neurourology and Urodynamics 13* (1994): 515–20; C. L. Parsons, M. Greenberger, L. Gabal, M. Bidair, G. Barme, and P. M. Hanno, "The Role of Urinary Potassium in the Pathogenesis and Diagnosis of Interstitial Cystitis," *Journal of Urology 159* (1998): 1862–66; discussion 1866–67.

2. C. L. Parsons, Jeffrey Dell, Edward J. Stanford, Michael Bullen, Bruce S. Kahn, and John J. Willems, "The Prevalence of Interstitial Cystitis in Gynecologic Patients with Pelvic Pain, as Detected by Intravesical Potassium Sensitivity," *American Journal of Obstetrics and Gynecology 187* (2002): 1395–400.

3. C. L. Parsons, Jeffrey Dell, Edward J. Stanford, Michael Bullen, Bruce S. Kahn, Tracy Waxell, and James A. Koziol, "Increased Prevalence of Interstitial Cystitis: Previously Unrecognized Urologic and Gynecologic Cases Identified Using a New Symptom Questionnaire and Intravesical Potassium Sensitivity," *Urology 60* (2002): 573–78.

BIBLIOGRAPHY

RESOURCES FOR PATIENTS

Beate Carrière, P. T., and P. T. Stuttgart. *Fitness for the Pelvic Floor.* New York: Thieme, 2002.

Cohen, Darlene. *Finding a Joyful Life in the Heart of Pain.* Boston: Shambhala, 2000.

Davies, Clair, and Amber Davies. *The Trigger Point Therapy Workbook—Your Self-treatment Guide for Pain Relief.* Oakland, CA: New Harbinger, 2004.

Egoscue, Pete, with Roger Gittines. *Pain Free for Women—The Revolutionary Program for Ending Chronic Pain.* New York: Bantam Books, 2002.

Glazer, Howard, and Gae Rodke. *The Vulvodynia Survival Guide: How to Overcome Painful Vaginal Symptoms and Enjoy an Active Lifestyle.* Oakland, CA: New Harbinger, 2002.

Hulme, Janet. *Pelvic Pain and Low Back Pain—A Handbook for Self Care and Treatment. 1st ed.* Missoula, MT: Phoenix, 2002.

International Association for the Study of Pain. "Global Year against Pain in Women—Real Women, Real Pain." http://www.iasp-pain.org/AM/Template.cfm?Section=Real_Women_Real_Pain&Template=/CM/HTMLDisplay.cfm&ContentID=4629.

Interstitial Cystitis Association. "Interstitial Cystitis and Pain—Taking Control—A Handbook for People with IC and Their Caregivers." Interstitial Cystitis Association. https://secure3.realssl.com/ichelp/store/shop.cgi?page=Topic07.html.

Kabat-Zinn, Jon. *Full Catastrophe Living—Using the Wisdom of Your Body and Mind to Face Stress, Pain, and Illness.* New York: Delta, 2005.

Kaysen, Susanna. *The Camera My Mother Gave Me.* New York: Alfred A. Knopf, 2001.

Maines, Rachel P. *The Technology of Orgasm: "Hysteria," the Vibrator, and Women's Sexual Satisfaction.* Baltimore: The Johns Hopkins University Press, 1999.

Moldwin, Robert M. *The Interstitial Cystitis Survival Guide.* Oakland, CA: New Harbinger, 2000.

Pausch, Randy, and Jeffrey Zaslow. *The Last Lecture.* New York: Hyperion, 2008.

Sadigh, Micah R. *Autogenic Training—A Mind-Body Approach to the Treatment of Fibromyalgia and Chronic Pain Syndrome.* New York: Haworth Medical Press, 2001.

Sokolove, Michael Y. *Warrior Girls—Protecting Our Daughters against the Injury Epidemic in Women's Sports.* New York: Simon and Schuster, 2008.

Sternberg, Esther M. *The Balance Within—The Science Connecting Health and Emotions.* New York: W. H. Freeman, 2000.

Villegas-Echeverri, Juan Diego, and Claudia Camila Giraldo-Parra. "Chronic Pelvic Pain Associated with the Bladder: We Know It Exists but How Should We Name It?" *IPPS Newsletter* 15, no. 4 (2008). http://www.pelvicpain.org/news/pdfs/vol15_no4.pdf.

RESOURCES FOR HEALTH CARE PROFESSIONALS

The following sources are geared toward the medical professional for the treatment and understanding of chronic pelvic/sexual pain. These are the best of the key works that address the full spectrum of understanding and managing chronic pelvic/sexual pain.

Beate Carrière, P. T., Cynthia Markel Feldt, and P. T. Stuttgart, eds. *The Pelvic Floor.* New York: Georg Thieme, 2006.

Berkley, K. J. "A Life of Pelvic Pain." *Physiology and Behavior* 86 (2005): 272–80.

Collett, B. J., C. J. Cordle, E. R. Stewart, and C. Jagger. "A Comparative Study of Women with CPP, Chronic Nonpelvic Pain and Those with No Physical Pain Attending General Practitioners." *British Journal of Obstetrics and Gynecology* 105 (1998): 87–92.

Howard, Fred. "Chronic Pelvic Pain." *Obstetrics and Gynecology* 103 (2004): 589–605.

Howard, Fred M., C. Paul Perry, James E. Carter, Ahmed M. El-Minawi, and Rong-Zeng Lie, eds. *Pelvic Pain: Diagnosis and Management.* Philadelphia: Lippincott Williams and Wilkins, 2000.

Mathias, S. D., M. Kuppermann, R. F. Liberman, R. C. Lipschutz, and J. F. Steege. "Chronic Pelvic Pain: Prevalence, Health-Related Quality of Life, and Economic Correlates." *Obstetrics and Gynecology* 87 (1996): 321–27.

Parsons, C. L. "The Role of the Urinary Epithelium in the Pathogenesis of Interstitial Cystitis/Prostatitis/Urethritis." *Urology* 69 (2007): S9–S16.

Parsons, C. L., Jeffrey Dell, Edward J. Stanford, Michael Bullen, Bruce S. Kahn, Tracy Waxell, and James A. Koziol. "Increased Prevalence of Interstitial Cystitis: Previously Unrecognized Urologic and Gynecologic Cases Identified Using a New Symptom Questionnaire and Intravesical Potassium Sensitivity." *Urology* 60 (2002): 573–78.

Parsons, C. L., C. Greenspan, and S. G. Mulholland. "The Primary Antibacterial Defense Mechanism of the Bladder." *Investigations in Urology* 13 (1975): 72–78.

Parsons, C. L., and V. Tatsis. "Prevalence of Interstitial Cystitis in Young Women." *Urology* 64 (2004): 866–70.

Steege, John F., Deborah A. Metzger, and Barbara S. Levy, eds. *Chronic Pelvic Pain: An Integrated Approach.* Philadelphia: Saunders, 1998.

Teichman, J. M., and C. L. Parsons. "Contemporary Clinical Presentation of Interstitial Cystitis." *Urology* 69 (2007): 41–47.

Thorn, Beverly E. *Cognitive Therapy for Chronic Pain: A Step-by-Step Guide.* New York: Guilford Press, 2004.

Wise, David, and Rodney Anderson. *A Headache in the Pelvis—A New Understanding and Treatment for Prostatitis and Chronic Pelvic Pain Syndromes.* Occidental, CA: National Center for Pelvic Pain, 2008.

Zondervan, K. T., P. L. Yudkin, M. P. Vessey, M. G. Dawes, D. H. Barlow, and S. H. Kennedy. "Patterns of Diagnosis and Referral in Women Consulting for Chronic Pelvic Pain in UK Primary Care." *British Journal of Obstetrics and Gynaecology* 106 (1999): 1156–61.

ONLINE RESOURCES

Secret Suffering Web Site

http://www.secretsuffering.com

Bladder—Painful Bladder Syndrome and Interstitial Cystitis

Interstitial Cystitis Association: http://www.ichelp.org
International Painful Bladder Association: http://www.painful-bladder.org
Interstitial Cystitis Network: http://www.ic-network.com

Lower Bowel

International Foundation for Functional Gastrointestinal Disorders: http://www.aboutibs.org

Pain

American Pain Foundation: http://www.painfoundation.org
American Pain Society: http://www.ampainsoc.org
International Pelvic Pain Society: http://www.pelvicpain.org
OBGYN.net's Pelvic Pain page: http://www.obgyn.net/pelvic-pain

Sexual Health

American Association of Sex Educators, Counselors, and Therapists: http://www.aasect.org
Information on Female Sexual Dysfunction: http://www.fsdinfo.org
Institute for Sexual Medicine, Boston University School of Medicine: http://www.bumc.bu.edu/sexualmedicine
National Institute of Health, National Library of Medicine: http://www.nlm.nih.gov/medlineplus/femalesexualdysfunction.html
Sexual Health Network: http://www.sexualhealth.com
Woman's Sexual Health Foundation: http://www.twshf.org

Vulvodynia

National Vulvodynia Association: http://www.nva.org

Vulvodynia.com: http://www.vulvodynia.com

Vulvodynia Web site in Poland:

(In Polish) http://www. vulvodynia.pl

(Translated to English) http://translate.google.com/translate?u=http%3A%2F%2Fwww.
    vulvodynia.pl&sl=pl&tl=en&hl=en&ie=UTF-8

INDEX

ABOUT THE AUTHORS

SUSAN BILHEIMER is a freelance and technical writer with eighteen years experience. Her articles and personality profiles have appeared in regional and national magazines, and her weekly column, *That's Life*, appeared in a series of Pennsylvania newspapers for over five years. Among her books are *How to Become a Technical Writer*, *Wandering Mind Meditation*, *Living with Sam*, *A Retreat of One's Own*, and the booklet *64 Tips to Relieve Sexual Pain*. In 2003, Bilheimer's interest in women's midlife issues led to the creation of an informational website on perimenopause (www.perimenopausesupport.com). Her own struggle with sexual and pelvic pain drove her to write *Secret Suffering*, and she developed the Secret Suffering website (www.SecretSuffering.com) to aid and support other women who live with this affliction.

ROBERT J. ECHENBERG, M.D., board certified in Obstetrics and Gynecology, is an established practitioner in the field of chronic pelvic/sexual pain in women. In 2001, after a 30 year career as an OB/GYN, basing his knowledge on experts in this rapidly developing field, he gradually developed a successful treatment model for this complex pain syndrome. Many hundreds of women (and even some men) have benefited from his program over the past eight years. He has spoken nationally and internationally on sexuality, medical ethics, and pelvic pain in women. Echenberg's private practice is located in Bethlehem, PA.